ID0938457

TOTAL QUALITY MANAGEMENT for HOME CARE

Elaine R. Davis, CPHQ
Examiner, Malcolm Baldrige National Quality Award
Since 1992

Chief Quality Officer
ASB Meditest
Framingham, Massachusetts

AN ASPEN PUBLICATION®

Aspen Publishers, Inc.
Gaithersburg, Maryland
1994

Library of Congress Cataloging-in-Publication Data

Davis, Elaine R.
Total quality management for home care / Elaine R. Davis
p. cm.
Includes bibliographical references and index.
ISBN 0-8342-0332-4
1. Home care services—Administration. 2. Total quality
management. I. Title.
[DNLM: 1. Home Care Services—organization & administration.
2. Quality of Health Care. WY 115 D261t]
RA645.3.D38 1992
362.1'4—dc20
DNLM/DLC
for Library of Congress
92-22048
CIP

Editorial Resources: Ruth Bloom

Library of Congress Catalog Card Number: 92-22048
ISBN: 0-8342-0332-4

Printed in the United States of America

1 2 3 4 5

This book has been many years in the making, and several people are responsible for its completion. I owe my personal thanks to Patricia Sanders, without whom I wouldn't have begun; to Vickie Trevarthan, who taught me more than I really wanted to know about infection control and assisted in the preparation of the audits; to Bruce Paulk, who pushed me all the way; but most of all, I owe a debt of gratitude and appreciation to all the employees, both past and present, of American Home Health Care, without whom this book would not be possible.

Table of Contents

Introduction

Some form of quality assurance has been around since 221 B.C., when the Chou Dynasty required physicians to pass exams before entering practice.[1] Because the health care profession has been unable to reach agreement on a definition of quality, little progress has been made in the quality discipline over the centuries. No real substantive work was done in the field until Ernest Codman devised the "end result system" between 1912 and 1916. This system was an evaluation of care based on the concept of outcome indicators.[2] Not until the Joint Commission on Accreditation of Healthcare Organizations (Joint Commission) adopted a medical audit program in the early 1970s did standards governing hospital accreditation begin to approach Codman's concepts.[3] However, by 1979, the Joint Commission acknowledged that the potential for audits to effect sustained improvement in patient care had been lost.

Government and other programs of quality assurance began to proliferate at this time. All of the programs talked about quality without defining it or developing any quantitative measure as to how to achieve it. One commentator has noted:

> Because salient indicators of quality of care are still elusive, it is virtually impossible to know the extent to which the models for the provision of health services and existing regulatory programs are working synergistically, antagonistically, or noninteractively to ensure appropriate quality of care.[4]

Clearly, a new approach was needed. In 1985, the Joint Commission introduced accreditation requirements for the development of quality and appropriateness of care monitoring and evaluation. Later this approach was extended to the home care industry. Home care had never before been considered formally in the quality continuum. Having survived its infancy, the home care industry is now emerging as the preferred provider of health services and, as such, is in a unique position to take the leadership role in the emergence of quality as a new medical discipline.

Today, health care professionals are beginning to hear concepts that heretofore have been within the exclusive purview of manufacturing and other industries. Concepts such as continuous quality improvement, statistical process control, and total quality management are emerging as the new frontier for the quality discipline. Hospitals are subjected to Joint Commission standards based on quality improvement. Additional new standards consistent with the expanded role of quality will be issued for home care as early as 1995. The concepts of continuous quality improvement, including statistical thinking and process control, will be incorporated into the Joint Commission's new standards. Since the concepts are new to all health care providers, home care for once need not be considered behind in the quest for quality.

Even though the home care industry has been the proverbial latecomer to the quality discipline, it has the opportunity to take the lead in developing new standards of quality. As an industry, home care has been in a reactive posture. As regulatory changes address quality, so too does home care. The industry as a whole has viewed the issue of quality assurance as one of conforming to the payer's rules and guidelines. Home care managers have considered quality to be a clinical function distinct from other operational issues. The decade of the 1990s will prove this old concept of quality to be defunct.

Quality in the home care agency of tomorrow will be a process that starts when the phone rings for an inquiry and proceeds long after the patient has been discharged. In the future, quality will incorporate the expectations of all customers, not just the payers. It will be expanded to every phase of the operation and will become an integral part of the overall business plan. Quality will become synonymous with customer satisfaction and will be the primary responsibility of the chief executive officer. It will be moved from the clinician's room to the boardroom.

This progressive movement of quality will be propelled by an increasingly knowledgeable consumer and fueled by regulatory environmental mandates. Competitive advantage will drive this movement and its parade will be national recognition through awards such as the Malcolm Baldrige National Quality Award.

Continuous quality improvement will provide the foundation for any agency to build an integrated quality program from which great achievement can be launched.

Please note that we have used the words "client" and "patient" interchangeably for ease of language and not necessarily to reflect the context.

NOTES

1. D.J. Fine and E.R. Meyer, *Quality Assurance in Historical Perspective* (Washington, D.C.: American Psychiatric Press, 1985).

2. E.A. Codman, *A Study in Hospital Efficiency: The First Five Years* (Boston: Thomas Todd & Company, 1916).

3. National Association of Quality Assurance Professionals, *Guide to Health Care Quality Management* (Deerfield, Ill.: National Association of Quality Assurance Professionals, 1991).

4. L.R. Tancredi, *Cost, Quality and Access in Health Care* (San Francisco: Jossey-Bass Publishers, 1988).

Chapter 1

The Quality Improvement Model for Home Care

Traditional thinking about concepts of quality no longer applies in today's highly competitive marketplace. The days when quality was considered only a clinical function, when management could delegate the assurance of quality to a director or a quality assurance committee, and when quality was "assumed" are over. Former President George Bush said, "The improvement of quality in products and the improvement of quality in service—these are national priorities as never before."[1] This quotation, which appeared on the front cover of the Malcolm Baldrige National Quality Award guidelines in 1991, emphasized today's thinking regarding the quality discipline.

Total quality management (TQM) is about doing business. It must be management led and customer oriented. Total quality is not just the latest management fad; it is a new way of thinking that will require fundamental changes in the way we do business.

> When it comes to improving what we do, there seems to be a flavor-of-the-month approach with each new, highly touted technique stepping on the heels of the one that went before—management by objective, management by results, management by problem report and resolution. Those are the cookbook methods, where you blend the worker and the machine, stir in a pinch of raw material, add a promise of a bonus (or a threat of dismissal), half-bake for 30 minutes and declare a dividend. It's easy to explain, easy to understand and it doesn't work.[2]

What does work, and has been working for over 50 years, is continuous quality improvement. This concept was first introduced to the Japanese after World War II by W. Edwards Deming. Prior to Deming's involvement with the Japanese, their products were cheap and had a reputation for poor quality. Today, Japanese quality is perceived as superior. Deming helped this transformation take place by showing the Japanese that quality had to be built into products and services.

Quality cannot be inspected into anything. If quality is not present at the end point of production (whether it's making a product or performing a service), the only choice management has is to rework, scrap, or start over. In home care, for example, if the plan of treatment was not done correctly the first time, it must be redone before it can be sent to the physician's office for signature. This is a costly proposition, yet it is the route most American businesses have taken. Deming demonstrated a better way—to look at the processes that produce goods and services and begin to understand them through statistical methods. Improvements should be based on data and focused on the customer. Employees have to be empowered to make the changes necessary to satisfy the customer and allowed to experience the pride of accomplishment.

The principles and concepts that transformed Japan and have been used for many years in industry are as applicable to the home care setting as they are to the manufacture of an automobile. This book will attempt to apply these proven techniques to the specifics of managing a home care agency.

The principles of continuous quality improvement (CQI) have been adopted universally. The International Standards Organization (ISO) has produced the ISO 9000–9004 Series of quality management and quality assurance standards. These standards are applicable to any organization doing business in the international market and speak to the issues of CQI. The Malcolm Baldrige National Quality Award is given by the President of the United States to companies that best exemplify quality improvements that have a sustained impact. Both the ISO standards and the Malcolm Baldrige standards are discussed in detail in subsequent chapters.

The Joint Commission has begun the transition to CQI. Standards incorporating the concepts of quality improvement have been applicable for hospitals since 1992 and will be applicable for home care by 1995. In a recent publication, the Joint Commission said

> This movement is adapting the philosophy and tools that industries have used to effectively improve the levels of quality in their products and services. If we can use the tools of continuous quality improvement to achieve greater efficiencies in the delivery of health care services, reduce costs, and improve quality, we will also have done much to reassert the private sector's leadership for quality in health care.[3]

Before we in the home care industry can begin to explore all of the advantages of CQI, we must build a firm foundation of surveillance and monitoring techniques to support and build a data base of reliable information. This book will address these issues in great detail. Many professionals have taken one of

W. Edwards Deming's 14 management points literally. Dr. Deming, in point 3, said to cease dependence on mass inspection. (See Chapter 2, Exhibit 2–1.) However, he goes on to say, use statistical methods to eliminate the need for mass inspection. Any process will deteriorate (worsen) without consistent monitoring. Having an objective basis for monitoring and surveillance activities is fundamental to process improvement. The place to begin on our road to continuously improved quality is with the board of directors and the senior managers. How many times have you heard, "Quality care is the most important thing in our agency." Yet, when you ask specifically, "How much money did your agency spend on quality last year?" typical answers vary from "I don't know" to "less than one percent of the corporate budget." If quality is so important, then why is so little money spent or why are the employees unaware of how much is being spent? Another key question is what is the cost of quality and the cost of nonquality? Without knowing these values, how can improvements be measured?

The board of directors should provide focus to the quality improvement program in accordance with the corporate vision. The most consistent problem encountered in developing a comprehensive approach to quality, assuming the vision speaks to this issue, is lack of focus. For example, most home care providers use some type of verification of billing before submitting claims to the intermediary. This is a valid audit process, but has nothing to do with the outcome of care rendered or the satisfaction of clients.

With the Medicare cost cap limitations juxtaposed to continually increasing nursing and other administrative costs, it becomes imperative that agencies utilize the little time and money they have available for monitoring activities that have the greatest impact on established outcome criteria. For example, every process has an outcome that should at least meet the requirements of customers of that process. The payroll process, for instance, has the check as an outcome or output with the primary customer being the employee. This focused approach should be evident in the agency's mission statement.

The board of directors of the home care agency should develop a compelling vision for the corporation that will serve as a basis for all services and functions. This vision, or mission statement, should be meaningful to the entire staff. A mission statement such as, ". . . meeting customer expectations in every service we provide," may be considered. Employees will need to "buy into" the vision in order to accomplish the mission. The following vision was developed by American Home Health Care in Atlanta, Georgia:

Enhancing quality of life through the delivery of compassionate health care at home by skilled professionals continuously striving for excellence.

The development of a corporate mission statement should not be taken lightly. The vision is the one thing that can bring all employees together in a common quest. If the corporate directors want to increase profitability, for example, employees probably are not going to get excited. On the other hand, employees can get excited over becoming the best home care agency or helping others to improve their quality of life. It is equally important that employees feel they have a part in developing the mission statement. After all, the employees, not the directors, will accomplish the quality goals.

Once the agency directors and employees agree on a mission statement, it will provide the focus necessary for all subsequent quality efforts. It is also important to recognize that quality is driven from the top down, not from the bottom up. In this regard, the board, president, administrator, and other senior leaders must see quality as a strategic imperative and integrate quality planning with overall business planning. This book will attempt to assist the agency in developing a focused approach to achieving quantifiable quality and continuously improving on that quality.

THE DEMING MODEL

The Deming model of quality and productivity[4] builds, in stages, a methodology for the process of quality. This method systematically approaches quality through definition, process, audit, and, ultimately, improvement. The model is found in Figure 1–1. What is quality? It has been said that defining quality is very much like defining pornography—we know what it is when we see it, but it's hard to define.[5] Many people talk about quality but do not take appropriate action to ensure the result. "Quality is never an accident—it is always the result of intelligent effort."[6]

Achieving quality is a process that results in attaining a desired or expected outcome. The Joint Commission has defined patient care quality as "the degree to which patient care services increase the probability of desired patient outcomes and reduce the probability of undesired outcomes, given the current state of knowledge." Given this definition, in order to improve quality, we must improve the outcomes of patient care interventions. In order to do so, we must have in place a monitoring system that addresses outcomes in a quantifiable manner.

Quality can be defined more universally as:

- conformance to requirements
- continued improvement toward excellence

For the purposes of this book, a generic definition of quality will be utilized— "consistent conformance to customer expectations with minimal variation."

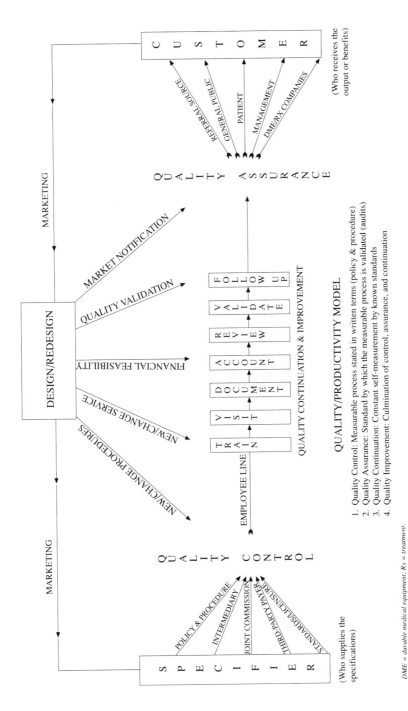

QUALITY/PRODUCTIVITY MODEL

1. Quality Control: Measurable process stated in written terms (policy & procedure)
2. Quality Assurance: Standard by which the measurable process is validated (audits)
3. Quality Continuation: Constant self-measurement by known standards
4. Quality Improvement: Culmination of control, assurance, and continuation

DME = durable medical equipment; Rx = treatment.

Note: Model modified from work of W. Edwards Deming—Japan Management, 1950.

Figure 1–1 Quality Productivity Model

In order for employees to conform to requirements or expectations, the employees must know what they are and have them in written form. The more aware the staff become of written expectations, the better the chances for improved performance that improves patient care outcomes. In fact, the meaning behind CQI is a continuous improvement in processes and requirements to better meet customer expectations. You cannot improve processes without a definition of the process or without clear, written instructions of the requirements.

Quality care includes four major components:

1. professional performance
2. efficient use of resources
3. minimal risk to the client of injury or illness associated with care
4. patient satisfaction

Each of these components can be found in the quality/productivity model. The model brings together the elements of quality care with efficiency and productivity. Caregivers must come to the realization that quality is synonymous with efficiency and productivity. Each is less effective without the other. Therefore, the model begins the process of quality with written controls that assist both managers and employees to understand expectations.

QUALITY CONTROL

Quality control is a measurable process that is stated in written terms usually seen as policies and procedures of an agency derived from the expectations of customers. The policies and procedures are a basic first step to ensuring quality, since they set forth expected behavior in conformance with stated customer expectations. Policies and procedures should be written in a format that clearly defines how the procedure is to be implemented. These procedures also should encompass the practice or protocol of the agency for a specific function. For example, some agencies change a central line dressing every 72 hours, while others change these dressings once a week. The procedure should define specifically the agency's expectations in lieu of a physician's specific order for the frequency of dressing change to the contrary.

It is important to remember that if one cannot measure, one cannot manage. For example, a policy statement may read, "It is the policy of the agency to provide the highest quality care for the lowest possible cost." This statement is laudable. However, it is not measurable, and therefore unenforceable or unmanageable. How do you know if you are meeting this objective or if you are doing better or worse without a quantifiable means to measure performance?

The statement could be changed to read, "It is the policy of this agency to ensure that nationally recognized standards of care are met or exceeded while maintaining costs at or below the federal limitation." In this example, the ambiguous "highest quality care" was changed to a measurable standard. Also changed was the unmeasurable "lowest possible cost" to a controlled cost that can be measured.

In addition to agency policies and procedures, quality control encompasses other "specifiers." A specifier is a group, either governmental or otherwise, that requires some level of performance from the services to be rendered. For example, a Medicare-certified agency must perform services under the federal Conditions of Participation, governed by the fiscal intermediary. The Joint Commission applies standards should an agency choose to go through the accreditation process. Third-party payers have certain guidelines or rules that must be followed for reimbursement. Those states that have licensure laws for home care impose rules under which an agency must operate. All of these groups are specifiers; each has its own set of rules and regulations.

Quality control is a proactive process whereby all the rules that must be followed are incorporated into a written measurable format and taught to those who render the care. Teaching caregivers is as important as committing the rules and regulations to paper. It is counterproductive to have the best policies, procedures, and other manuals if those rendering care do not know the information contained therein. Staff development is the key ingredient to successful internalization of the quality control standards.

As mentioned previously, the improvements necessary in health care will come from improvements in processes and requirements. Requirements, in the form of policy or procedure, are often written in broad, ambiguous terms. To improve performance of a requirement, it must be written in a manner that everyone who reads it will interpret the same way. For example, if I ask 3 out of 200 people to count the blue shirts in a room, chances are I will get 3 different answers. If I improve the requirements by asking them to count the men wearing solid blue shirts, I may now get 2 out of 3 correct answers. If I further improve my requirements by asking them to count the men wearing solid navy blue shirts, I may now get all 3 correct answers. Specificity of requirements is absolutely critical to assurance of desired performance.

QUALITY ASSURANCE

The second phase in the model is the quality assurance (QA) process. QA is one of the most misunderstood quality processes, simply because most providers believe it encompasses everything necessary to achieve quality. Such is not the case. QA is only one process in the quest to achieve optimum outcomes for clients.

QA is the standard by which the measurable process specified in quality control is validated. In other words, QA is a retroactive monitoring process. Like most audits, QA is performed after the fact. Audit results can be evaluated to determine whether standards were met. Knowledge is acquired more through the recognition of error than through the accumulation of new facts.[7] It is the goal of this book to demonstrate for the reader the necessity of finding and eliminating errors before they happen. When errors do happen, however, an attempt should be made to demonstrate how to recognize the error and correct it in order to improve the overall outcomes. The entire program of quality assurance and improvement should not be an inspection system. One cannot inspect quality into the service. Quality can only be built in.

At a recent meeting of the National Pathologist Association, one physician responded to a reporter's question by saying, "The pathologist is the best quality assurance mechanism in the hospital." This statement points out again the ultimate futility of finding errors after they happen.

This is not to say, however, that QA audits are unproductive. These audits play a key role in finding and noting trends for improvement opportunities so that corrective action to change, performance behaviors, or processes can be taken. The key to the success of QA audits is in the follow-up corrections made to processes and requirements and the subsequent training or retraining of staff. Figure 1–2 is offered as an illustration.

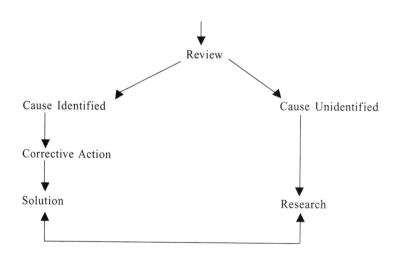

Figure 1–2 Review Cycle

Research or the discovery of new facts is necessary to overcome clinical impressions. For example, every agency director of nurses would undoubtedly say that all nurses on staff comply with sterile technique in the insertion of Foley catheters. However, if urinary tract infections (UTIs) are a consistent problem in the agency, a QA or infection control audit would be appropriate to determine the cause. Gathering data from such research or review is the only method to dispel the mistaken clinical impression. Frequently, agency administrators or department managers rely far too heavily on their own presumptions or what others have told them, without any means of validation. In the case of consistent UTIs, a research project or audit of catheter insertion technique could reveal the root cause of this problem. Quality improvement is founded on management by fact, not presumptions.

There are a number of different types of QA audits or surveillance tools. Because of the variety of audits and the time needed to go through the audit process, it is important that agency personnel prioritize surveillance activities in order of importance or impact on patient care outcomes. The outcomes expected should also be stated as measures of performance (thresholds).

For example, a diagnosis-related audit will test a nurse's adherence to nationally recognized standards of care (aspects) that are designed to achieve specific patient outcomes based on a nursing intervention and that can be measured as indicators. If a nurse does not comply with these standards, the patient may not achieve optimum results. Therefore, this type of audit is of utmost importance.

On the other hand, an audit for the purpose of validating the number of visits billed will not have a direct impact on a patient's outcome criteria. This type of audit is important for reimbursement purposes but may not be assigned a high priority if the agency has limited resources to expend on quality assurance and improvement. However, if the agency has lost its Medicare waiver status or is having difficulties with insurance companies denying payment for services, a utilization review (UR) audit may become a high priority.

In order to determine appropriate priorities for QA surveillance, the following breakdown of types of audits is offered:

1. Type 1—QA—an audit process by which professional practice is validated utilizing nationally recognized standards of care by diagnosis or disease state.

2. Type 2—UR—an audit process by which appropriate utilization of services, including efficient use of resources and visits, is validated in accordance with guidelines established by payer source.

3. Type 3—Field Review—an audit process by which appropriate clinical technique is validated on the basis of standards of care in the home setting.

4. Type 4—Administrative Review—an audit process by which the clinical record, operational processes, or both are validated in accordance with established policies and procedures of the agency.

QA surveillance is costly and time consuming. Therefore, any audit undertaken should have a clearly defined purpose and scope with defined indicators that are related to improved patient outcomes or another improvement opportunity. Audits must have a clear focus with no duplication in other audits. Above all, audits should be objective in nature. In other words, regardless of who performs the audit, the results should be the same. This recalls the "blue shirt" example given earlier. How many times have you seen medical record audits differ, based on who performed them? We often hear, "She is a hard auditor" or, "She is a tough auditor." These are examples of a misconception in the audit process. The problem in this scenario is that the audit process is flawed. The audit's requirements, scope, sources of data, indicators, or something in the audit process or tool is not specific enough to ensure consistent feedback. Therefore, the audit is vulnerable to subjective interpretation.

The objectivity of an audit is the most difficult goal to accomplish. For example, a question on an audit might read, "Are skilled services appropriate?" This question requires a judgment by the nurse conducting the audit. The judgment could be based on several variables:

- diagnosis
- patient's overall condition
- parameters of fluctuations in patient's condition
- length of stay
- competency of patient or caretaker
- physician orders
- home environment

Because of all these variables, one nurse may say skilled services are appropriate and another may say they are not. This lack of specificity is confusing to the field staff who want to do it right the first time but need to know exactly what "right" is and how it will be judged. Therefore, indicators used as criteria on the QA audit should be based on fact, either documented or observed. Questions should be worded to elicit a response that is not subject to a judgment call. Words such as "appropriate" are subject to interpretation and should be avoided.

In more advanced QA systems, judgment can be used where that judgment is based on specified and measurable parameters. In these systems, computers are often used for scoring because of the complexity involved. Each parameter or indicator is point-scored, and the computer makes the determination. For example, the question on an audit tool may be, "Were the number of visits appropriate to the diagnosis?" Preset parameters would be point-scored based on importance level; i.e., condition status, vital sign ranges, complicating variables, presence or absence of caregiver, contributing diagnoses, etc. Little computer programming work has been done in this area other than that done by accreditation groups. Agencies can, however, develop an audit tool for QA based on identifying the contributors to care outcomes that will result in the greatest probability for improved patient care.

Much has been said regarding the role of QA in health care in light of the more progressive CQI techniques. Many would have us believe that QA is passé. Nothing is further from the truth. The confusion may be from point 3 of Deming's 14 management points that says, ". . . cease dependence on mass inspection." Deming is not against performing QA activities. He has only maintained that you cannot rely upon QA activities as the *sole* means of assuring quality. Deming teaches that we must never be devoid of information about how the system is performing. This is clearly a QA function that will change in the CQI environment, to be sure, but must continue to provide information to management on how the patient care process is performing. The QA role, as outlined here, moves QA from the old subjective model to an objective, quantifiable model that will support quality improvement initiatives.

QUALITY CONTINUATION

The third phase in the quality system is continuation. This phase deals exclusively with constant self-measurement by known standards and is proactive. The known standards come from the specifiers under the quality control phase that have been taught and reinforced with field and other staff. In other words, staff must be able to measure their own performance by standards they not only know but have internalized.

Once a standard is internalized, it becomes second nature or overlearned and is practiced without the cognitive thought process. For example, a nurse will walk into the patient's room and begin assessing while saying good morning. This is the process of internalization of learned behavior. When the staff can internalize the standards so thoroughly that the expected behavior becomes routine, then the process of self-evaluation by known standards becomes routine and the continuation of quality is achieved.

Quality continuation is the alignment of quality policy, procedure, practice, hiring criteria, training, rewards, and recognition. It is about "walk-the-talk." For example, if management stresses compliance with Occupational Safety and Health Administration (OSHA) standards but does not provide biohazardous containers or other necessary equipment to fully comply, there is a disconnect between the words and the action. The staff must see alignment between what management says and does for effective quality continuation.

If quality improvement is important to the agency, then training in these techniques is necessary for the entire staff. Policies and procedures will have to be rewritten in specific, quantifiable terms. Acceptable quality levels will have to give way to continuous improvement in patterns of practice, and the staff will know what management considers to be important by the way employees are rewarded and recognized.

The first step toward an empowered work force is to develop the means by which the staff can measure its performance in accordance with known, quantifiable standards. Today's measurement systems need to be reevaluated in light of the more quantifiable methods of CQI. These methods will be discussed in more detail in subsequent chapters.

Staff development plays a major role in quality continuation. Constant reinforcement of quality standards builds expectations into the service and those rendering care. The audit process inspects—but only the staff can accomplish the goal of conformance to quality standards on a consistent basis or identify process problems that create a barrier to improved care. The fundamental principle that quality must be built in as the service is rendered can only be applied by the staff rendering care. Expectations are for staff to behave in a certain way. Once this goal is accomplished, the final phase of quality is assured.

QUALITY IMPROVEMENT

The fourth and final phase in the process of quality management is that of improvement. This phase is the culmination of all other components and is the goal of all agencies.

Quality improvement does not just happen. It is the end result of developing the controlling standards, implementing the QA activities, and continuing to build quality by staff. It can be both proactive and retroactive. Improvement is not a constant; therefore, changes are frequent. Quality is a moving target and the "bar" will continue to be raised by a public with ever-higher expectations for health care delivery. Statistical tools are available to assist staff in the improvement effort. If agencies continue to do things today the way they did things yesterday, they will not be prepared to do new things tomorrow.

The health care field is constantly changing, and professionals must be prepared to keep pace with technology. The key to success is to stay high on the learning curve throughout the professional career. As the acceptable threshold of a given standard is achieved, the time has come to raise the threshold to higher levels for more improvement.

For example, assume an outcome threshold is to achieve 80 percent compliance with demonstrated return on teaching new diabetic patients. Also assume this percentage is consistently achieved throughout the agency. Given this set of circumstances, the threshold should be raised to 85 or 90 percent compliance, thus pushing for improvement. Specific outcome criteria and thresholds will be discussed in detail in subsequent chapters.

When technology changes or when a new service is offered, the process begins over with new quality control standards, a QA surveillance process, teaching with constant reinforcement to achieve quality improvement, and continuous improvements to processes. This process is called design or redesign.

In the quality/productivity model, improvement can be suggested from several sources. We have discussed the opportunity to improve internal thresholds. Another source of quality improvement can come from the agency's customers. It is important that the health care provider realize that there is a direct relationship between the customer and quality. This relationship may only be perceived; that is, if the customer is satisfied with care, the quality has been achieved.

The customer must be satisfied with care or there will not be a perception of quality, regardless of whether all standards were in compliance. There are two types of quality: quality by perception and quality in fact. Most patients do not know if the care or procedure was technically correct. The decision regarding quality is dependent almost entirely on patient perception of the caregiver during the interaction. On the other hand, a physician is in a position to determine the technical accuracy of a procedure based on its outcome. These two types of quality carry equal weight and both must be addressed within the quality system. Customer satisfaction ratings are therefore an important component in quality improvement. If ratings are lower than expected, the agency would need to review, through the design or redesign process, why customers are not satisfied. This process is fully discussed later in this text.

Additionally, if a customer is a physician who serves hemophiliacs, the physician may request the agency to do blood transfusions in the home. It cannot be emphasized enough that an agency should *not* attempt to provide any new service or products without going through each phase of quality as identified in Figure 1–1. To do so invites uncertainty, confusion, and potential harm to the patient.

There has been much literature on the subject of reengineering. Reengineering is a quality tool to design or redesign a process in compliance with stated or implied customer expectations and specifications. The methods used in reengineering are varied but all have the same basic components as found in the Deming quality and productivity model. Specifications and expectations come from the customers or users of the process. These are turned into requirements and operational definition in the design phase, and are subsequently taught to the staff complete with a self-measurement tool. The entire process is then validated through QA with adjustments made accordingly.

Alignment of human resource objectives is linked directly to the outcomes specified or expected by the customers. This closes the "quality loop" and provides the impetus for customer-driven quality. These concepts will be discussed in detail in Chapter 4.

Process reengineering begins with a complete understanding of the current status of the operation or process to be redesigned or improved. This should include a flowchart and the operational definitions currently in use. The next step is to conduct customer-based research to determine the satisfaction level with current practices and to what extent changes should be made. The research will also determine the key quality characteristics of the process or the most important attributes of customer service that should be met consistently. The design of a research tool will be discussed in Chapter 4.

Next, the process is designed to consistently meet the customer's expectations. This becomes an exercise in "how-to". For example, research reveals that customers want physical therapy to begin on new cases within 24 hours of admission to the agency. How will a system be designed that will ensure the agency can deliver on this key service attribute? The process used to consistently meet customer expectations is one of the most important in reengineering. There are a number of advanced quality tools available for this purpose, such as quality function deployment (QFD). However, for the beginner, brainstorming, fishbone diagramming, and other basic tools can be used effectively. These tools are discussed in subsequent chapters.

The next step in process design or redesign is to add value through a method called *value analysis.* While this method is usually employed by the more advanced users of the quality sciences, it can be used by beginners through the simple tools discussed later in this text. The purpose of value analysis is to ensure that every step in the process adds value for the customer. If no value is added for the customer, then the step or task should be deleted. The deletion of no- or low-value tasks simplifies process and allows staff more time to concentrate on the key service attributes.

After determining the key service attributes or characteristics of a process and designing a method to consistently deliver it, the next step is creating the standard of performance. The performance standard will become the self-measurement vehicle by which the staff determines its level of conformance. This standard also gives the staff the opportunity to exceed the stated or implied expectations.

Home care is prime ground for Murphy's Law: if it can go wrong, it will! The next step in reengineering is to recognize where failure points are and design the process to prevent these failures. This step follows the development of the measurement system because often, the failure is in the measurement system itself. As previously noted, standards, processes, audits, procedures, and other protocols of performance have been written in a way that ensures varying responses. The improvement in processes is dependent on improvement in requirements.

When failure points have been designed out of the system, the new process or procedure must be completely documented. A good starting point is a flowchart of the process, followed by operational definitions. An operational definition is the specific, detailed procedural guide for performing each step in the process. These definitions should not be ambiguous or subject to interpretation.

The final step in design for process improvement is perhaps the most important. It is the link between what the customers want, how to provide it, who will provide it, and what the compensation will be for providing it. This final step closes the quality loop. In this step, job requirements and competencies, as well as the reward and recognition system, are defined. Figure 1–3 depicts the reengineering process.

If a new service or product is needed by the referral source, the agency should go through each phase of quality in a test mode before making the new service available to the general public. Remember that quality is never an accident—it is always the result of intelligent effort.

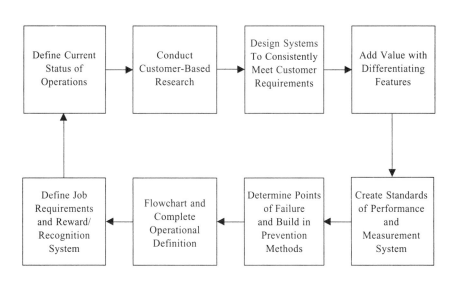

Figure 1–3 Reengineering Process

ORGANIZATIONAL STRUCTURE

The organizational structure for quality improvement has six components or departments. In the more mature TQM environments, additional departments such as research and development as well as marketing could become a part of this structure. See Figure 1–4.

This organizational framework allows for optimum cooperation and facilitates the teamwork approach necessary to develop and maintain a prevention-based strategy for quality improvement. Functional responsibilities are as follows:

- Quality assurance
  1. audits (primary)
  2. Joint Commission compliance
  3. standards compliance
  4. licensure compliance
  5. state and federal regulations compliance
- Utilization review
  1. intermediary liaison
  2. client advocate with insurance company
- Risk management
  1. workers' compensation
  2. incident reporting
  3. occurrence reports
  4. OSHA reporting
- Infection control
  1. precautions
  2. waste disposal
  3. employee exposure
- Staff development
  1. orientation
  2. training (primary)
  3. preceptor program
  4. staff development programs
  5. levels program
- Customer service
  1. internal questionnaires
  2. external questionnaires
  3. market surveys
  4. postdischarge follow-up program
  5. client advocacy with agency and government

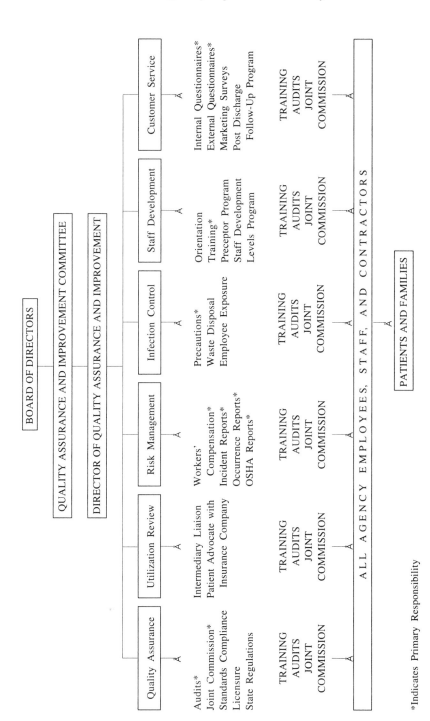

Figure 1–4 Quality Assurance and Improvement Model Organizational Structure

*Indicates Primary Responsibility

Each of the specific functions of these divisions will be discussed in detail in the following chapters. The point of departmentalizing the functions is to acknowledge their unique interrelationship to all other aspects of quality assurance and improvement. By departmentalizing these functions, specific responsibility can be assigned. When responsibility is assigned, so is accountability. For smaller agencies, the functions can be combined. When there is any doubt regarding the priority of a function, let the overriding goal of prevention be the guide. Throughout this book, prevention of error and opportunities for improvement are the cornerstones of the quality discipline.

Another way of looking at the organizational structure for the quality system is to organize around categories of issues. This approach has worked well in mature quality improvement environments. The improvement activities are grouped into seven major categories:

1. leadership and culture
2. strategic quality planning
3. information and analysis
4. process management and improvement
5. human resources planning and utilization
6. customer relationship management
7. quality and performance results

This level of organizational structure is cross-functional and involves every aspect of the agency and its leadership. As an agency develops its quality improvement initiatives, this approach should be considered. For beginners, however, the suggested approach is shown in Figure 1–4. This higher-level approach assumes the agency wants to achieve a world-class level of quality. (See Figure 1–5.) An example of a mission statement driving such an organization would be: "To exceed customer expectations in every service provided without exception."

A brief synopsis of each of these categories follows:

Leadership and Culture. The senior management's success in creating quality values and building these into operations.

Strategic Quality Planning. The agency's effective integration of the customer's quality requirements into the business plan.

Information and Analysis. The agency's effective collection and analysis of information for quality.

Process Management and Improvement. Process management must improve requirements, standards, and measures in order to constantly enhance the

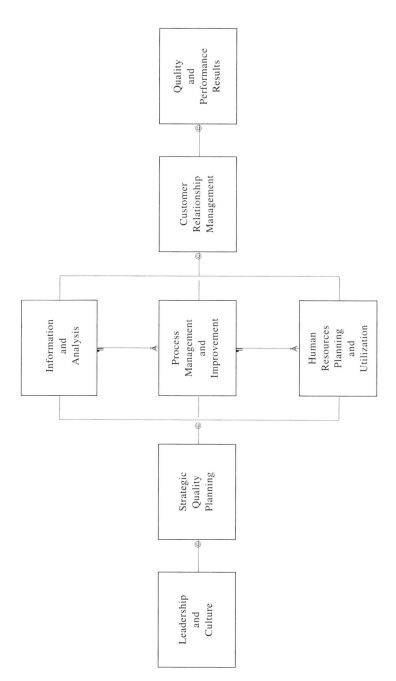

Mission: To Exceed Customer Expectations in Every Service We Provide without Exception

Figure 1–5 Continuous Quality Improvement Approach to World Class

organization's ability to exceed customer expectations in every service provided.

Human Resources Planning and Utilization. The success of the agency in realizing the full potential of the work force for quality.

Customer Relationship Management. The effectiveness of the agency's systems in determining customer requirements and demonstrated success in meeting them.

Quality and Performance Results. The agency's improvements in quality and demonstration of quality excellence based upon quantitative measures.

The above categories clearly demonstrate that this type of structure will require a high level of personnel—one with extensive training in the quality sciences. This approach is clearly more focused on the overall organization as opposed to the caregiving component of operations. However, care rendered is still the core business for home care agencies and as such must continue to be the focus of quality improvement activities. Figure 1–5 shows the cross-functional structure approach to world-class quality.

NOTES

1. National Institute for Standards and Technology, *Malcolm Baldrige National Quality Award* (1991), front cover.

2. L. Dobyns, Ed Deming Wants Big Changes and He Wants Them Fast, *Smithsonian* (August, 1990).

3. Joint Commission on Accreditation of Healthcare Organizations, *Using CQI Approaches To Monitor, Evaluate and Improve Quality Transitions from QA to QI* (Oakbrook, Ill.: JCAHO, 1991).

4. W. Edwards Deming, *The Quality/Productivity Model* (Japan Management, 1950).

5. International Conference on Quality Assurance, The Netherlands, attributed to Dr. Martin Bockboldt, May, 1989.

6. "Quality Is Never an Accident," paraphrased from Willa H. Foster.

7. McIntyre and Popper, *British Medical Journal* (1984).

Chapter 2

Continuous Quality Improvement

Quality improvement is a prevention-based strategy encompassing all of the agency's activities, not just clinical, and focuses squarely on the customer.

A commitment to quality can become the foundation for growth, will minimize risks, and allow for a greater retention of competent staff. Improvement of quality is an investment in the future of the agency.

Much has been written on the subject of quality recently. With the growth in popularity of the Malcolm Baldrige National Quality Award, business and industry have jumped on the bandwagon of quality in an all-out effort to meet foreign competition head on. Quality has been hailed as the "Holy Grail" of business and has moved from the back room to the boardroom. For the first time in history, manufacturing and other industrialized business and the providers of health care are all saying the same things—and using the same tools to accomplish the objectives! We are today in the midst of an exciting quality revolution that will propel us into the 21st century.

What happened to cause all this excitement? Continuous quality improvement (CQI) has been proven to accomplish all of the business and financial objectives traditionally viewed as the benchmarks of success. A U.S. General Accounting Office study rated Baldrige Award finalists on overall company performance attributable to quality programming. This landmark study revealed the following[1]:

> Market Share and Profitability: Performance indicators were market share, sales per employee, return on assets, and return on sales. Market share showed the most notable increase with companies reporting an average increase of 13.7 percent.[2]

Note: The author wishes to thank Professor Lawrence S. Aft, PE, for his enormous help in the preparation of this chapter.

Customer Satisfaction: Performance indicators were overall customer satisfaction, number of complaints, and customer retention. Customer satisfaction showed an annual average increase of 2.5 percent.

Quality and Cost: Performance indicators were reliability, timeliness of delivery, order processing time, errors or defects, product lead time, inventory turnover, costs of quality, and cost savings. Reliability improved by an annual average of 11.3 percent, order processing time was reduced by an annual average of 12 percent, and the average annual reduction in errors was 10.3 percent.

Employee Relations: Performance indicators were number of employee suggestions, employee satisfaction, attendance, turnover, and safety and health. The total number of suggestions showed the largest improvements going up by an average of 16.6 percent annually.

These striking results have proven that quality pays off in increased profitability, productivity, and competitive position while the overall cost of quality decreases. It is interesting to note that of all the important indicators of quality improvement, customer satisfaction improved the least (2.5 percent annual average) in the study. This may be a misnomer since the study was based on companies with a high degree of quality evidenced by their status in third-stage review under the Malcolm Baldrige National Quality Award. These companies already possessed a high degree of customer satisfaction to be able to advance that far in the Baldrige process. Concentrated efforts are generally not placed where there already is a high degree of satisfaction. Figure 2–1 illustrates the effects of continuous improvement.

THE GURUS

The concepts of CQI are very different from traditional quality assurance (QA) in the health care field. Some use CQI and total quality management (TQM) interchangeably. These concepts have their basis in industrial engineering and were first articulated by the quality gurus:

Dr. W. Edwards Deming. By far the most widely read and accepted of the gurus, Deming is credited with the CQI movement. He was responsible in the 1950s for training Japanese management in the field of statistical control of quality and is recognized by the Japanese Union of Scientists and Engineers

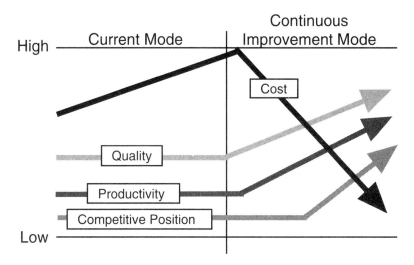

Figure 2–1 The Effects of Quality Improvement. *Source:* Adapted from QualPro seminar, 1990, results confirmed by GAO Study of Quality.

(JUSE) with the much coveted "Deming Prize." This prize has become the international symbol of quality and has been won only once by an American company, Florida Power and Light. Deming defines quality as "Continually meeting customers' needs and expectations at a price they are willing to pay." Deming's 14 Management Points is in wide use today in some of the world's most successful companies. (A copy of Deming's 14 points appears in Exhibit 2–1.)

Dr. Deming's most notable contribution to the quality sciences is his statistical work in defining process performance variability in terms of either special or common causes. Special causes are considered the responsibility of an individual employee and happen, according to Deming, only 6 percent of the time. Common causes, on the other hand, occur 94 percent of the time and are management's responsibility to correct. The significance of this hypothesis launched the movement that is known today as CQI.

The realization that poor process outcomes could not be blamed on individuals led to a revolution in QA that continues today. This revolution has changed the impetus from individual performance, where blame was attached, to the overall system's performance for improved outcomes. Deming's work has become the foundation upon which most quality improvement systems are based.

Dr. Joseph M. Juran. Juran's work expanded Deming's original work to include traditional management functions. Juran is perhaps best known for the

Exhibit 2-1 Deming's 14 Management Points

1. Create constancy of purpose toward improvement of product and service with a plan to become competitive, stay in business, and provide jobs.
2. Adopt the new philosophy. We are in a new economic age. We can no longer live with commonly accepted levels of delays, mistakes, defects, and poor workmanship.
3. Cease dependence on mass inspection. Require, instead, statistical evidence that quality is built in to eliminate the need for inspection on a mass basis.
4. End the practice of awarding business on the basis of price tag. Instead, depend on meaningful measures of quality along with price. Move toward a single supplier for any one item, on a long term relationship of loyalty and trust.
5. Improve constantly and forever the system of production and service, to improve quality and productivity, and thus constantly decrease costs.
6. Institute training on the job using modern training methods.
7. Institute leadership. The aim of leadership should be to help people do a better job.
8. Drive out fear, so that everyone may work effectively for the company.
9. Break down organizational barriers—everyone must work as a team to foresee and solve problems.
10. Eliminate arbitrary numerical goals, posters, and slogans for the work force which seek new levels of productivity without providing the methods.
11. Replace management by numbers with never-ending improvement.
12. Remove barriers that rob employees of their pride of workmanship.
13. Institute a vigorous program of education, training, and self-improvement.
14. Create a structure which will push the prior 13 points everyday. Transform the organization.

Source: Gitlow, H., and Gitlow, S., *The Deming Guide to Quality and Competitive Position,* Prentice-Hall, 1987.

Juran trilogy, made up of components of effective quality management. These are:

1. quality planning
2. quality control
3. quality improvement

Juran defines quality as "fitness for use." More specifically, he states that a product or service must be free of deficiencies or errors. The product must also meet the customer's perceived needs. A further explanation of the Juran trilogy appears in Exhibit 2-2.

Juran's work concentrates on the concept of building quality into the process from the beginning. His work in process design and engineering has proven foundational to what has become known as process reengineering.

Exhibit 2-2 The Juran Trilogy

QUALITY PLANNING	QUALITY CONTROL	QUALITY IMPROVEMENT
Determine who the customers are	Evaluate actual service performance	Establish the infrastructure
Determine the needs of the customers	Compare actual performance to service goals	Identify the improvement projects
Develop service features that respond to customers' needs	Act on the difference	Establish project teams
Develop processes able to produce the service features		Provide the teams with resources, training, and motivation to:
Transfer the plans to the operational divisions		• diagnose the causes • stimulate remedies • establish controls to hold the gains

Source: Adapted with permission of the Free Press, a Division of Macmillan, Inc., from *Juran on Leadership for Quality* by J.M. Juran. © 1989 by Juran Institute, Inc.

Philip Crosby. Crosby defines TQM as a strategic, integrated management system for achieving customer satisfaction that involves all managers and employees and uses quantitative methods to continuously improve an organization's processes.[3]

Crosby's contribution to quality improvement is described in his book, *Quality Is Free,* and is known as his "zero defects" concept. He, like the other gurus, believes that the definition of quality is "conformance to requirements."

Crosby also articulated four "quality absolutes":

1. The definition of quality is conformance to requirements.
2. The system of quality is prevention.
3. The performance standard is zero defects.
4. The measurement of quality is the price of nonconformance.

It is Crosby's work in the area of quality costing that brought him the greatest recognition. Crosby first articulated the cost of quality concepts that are used today in comprehensive quality systems. Crosby discussed quality in a universally understood term: money. The quantification of quality in financial terms propelled management to understand that it is cheaper to achieve quality than it is not to achieve it. Crosby divided quality costs into the following categories:

1. Prevention: Costs associated with preventing failures and quality problems. An example is training in quality control techniques.
2. Appraisal: Costs associated with achieving the desired levels of quality. Statistical process control is an example.
3. Internal failure: Costs associated with catching errors before they reach the customer. An example is the review of the plan of treatment (POT) before it is submitted to the physician.
4. External failure: Costs associated with errors that reach customers. An example is a denial. Other examples are catastrophic failures resulting in lawsuits, workers' compensation losses, and write-offs.

Crosby separated these categories into the price of conformance and the price of nonconformance. His work indicated that the smallest amount of resources are spent on prevention, which causes the enormous expenditures on nonconformance.

There are many other gurus who have contributed to the body of knowledge that comprises the quality sciences. Deming, Juran, and Crosby, however, forged the basic concepts underlying all quality systems.

It is clear from this overview of the quality gurus that, although each has a little different twist on the subject, they all basically agree on the principles. The definition of quality put forth in the first chapter of this book is consistent with the teachings of the gurus and will serve the home care industry well. To repeat the definition of quality: "Consistent conformance to customer expectations with minimal variation."

Reducing variation is the objective of quality improvement. Reduction of variation is not familiar to the home care industry. It involves consistency in the output of the process, based on established targets. For example, medication errors represent a variation from the norm. Any problem, by virtue of its deviation from standards or protocols, is a variation from the target. The "hows" of problem resolution or continuous improvements, after a problem has been resolved, can best be answered by quantitative, objective measures. Each of the gurus tell us that statistical data and tools can offer the most effective means of problem resolution for sustainable improvements.

Sustained improvements are the measure by which quality improvement tools and techniques are judged. The Hawthorne principle is a concept that was developed at the Hawthorne plant of Bell Labs. Quality and productivity were studied and a variety of techniques were tested. The end result was that no matter what tool, technique, method, or resource was used, the problem would improve as long as management paid attention to it. As soon as management diverted its attention from the situation, the situation would regress to the original state that created the problem. This principle functions exactly the same in a home care agency. If management pays careful attention to a problem, the problem improves. As soon as management relaxes its attention, the problem returns.

Sustained improvements defy the Hawthorne principle. Quality improvement tools and techniques have been designed to address not the symptoms, but the root cause of problems. They have been designed to address process problems, not people problems. They integrate all components of a quality system to effectively change the outcome to a more desirable state. If improvements can be sustained, and have been driven from a predefined approach, they can be replicated from one location to another.

The ability to effectively replicate a sustained improvement in a different location is the result of a quality improvement system. More details on the planning for this goal will be discussed in Chapter 3.

CQI CONCEPTS

The statistical tools for limiting variation and thereby improving quality came to the health care industry from the manufacturing environment, where these methods were tested and found to be the key to sustained improvements. Before the tools are introduced some basic concepts of quality improvement should be examined:

- Every problem has a root cause based in either a system or process.
- Every process (or system) has a distinct organizational flow and specified decision points for alternative actions or behaviors.
- Every process in health care (either clinical or administrative) has an upstream and downstream customer who will determine quality at the point of interface.
- Every process generates or produces some output that can be either measured or counted. (For example, a patient's blood pressure can be measured. On the other hand, medication errors can be counted.)
- Every process has a pattern or shape that is discernable when viewed in graphic form. This shape becomes the basis for all statistical studies and improvement efforts and is commonly referred to as the bell-shaped curve.
- Every process will have variation. Variation is a natural state but is the enemy of quality.
- Every process has key quality characteristics that add value for the downstream customer upon which standards can be set.
- Functions which do not add value for the downstream customer add waste cost to the agency.

TOOLS FOR ACHIEVING CQI

Specific tools can be utilized to assist in achieving the goals of continuous quality improvement. Each of the tools and techniques will be discussed where it applies within the context of the CQI concept. Before going into detail on these tools, it should be noted that the tools and techniques are to assist the user in improving quality. They are not an end unto themselves. The tools should not be considered the only means to improve quality, although they have been proven not only to improve quality but also to sustain the improvement.

Some quality professionals become so involved in the use of the techniques that they lose sight of their purpose. Simplicity is always best. Use the easiest tools for the purpose needed. As proficiency grows, more complex tools can be utilized. For purposes of this text, only basic quality improvement tools will be discussed.

Concept 1

Every problem has a root cause based in either a system or process.

This concept has created a great deal of difficulty for the home care industry. Health care providers have been taught from the beginning of their careers to place blame for problems. An enormous amount of time is spent tracking individuals to determine if they are to blame for quality deficiencies. When the surveyor cites the agency for untimely aide supervisory visits, nurses are blamed for inappropriate conduct.

The typical problem-solving paradigm is illustrated in Figure 2–2 and is another validation of the Hawthorne principle. Problems are temporarily solved as long as they are watched. Often, temporary solutions create another problem elsewhere. For example, while concentrating on conducting high quality aide supervisory visits in a timely manner, something else such as the care plan might slip.

The reason for this cycle of chronic problems is the failure to address the root cause of the problem. As Deming said, only 6 percent of the time will problems be caused by an individual or group of individuals. The problems actually lie in the root cause found in the system or process. Deming attributed systemic causes to 94 percent of all problems.

The root cause is deeper than it appears on the surface. People are generally thought to be the obvious cause of problems, but people actually only reflect the symptoms of the real cause. The Japanese have a game they play to determine the root cause of a problem. They ask "why" at least five times. Figure 2–3 illustrates the point for root cause.

Concept 2

Every process or system has a distinct organizational flow with specific decision points for alternative actions or behaviors.

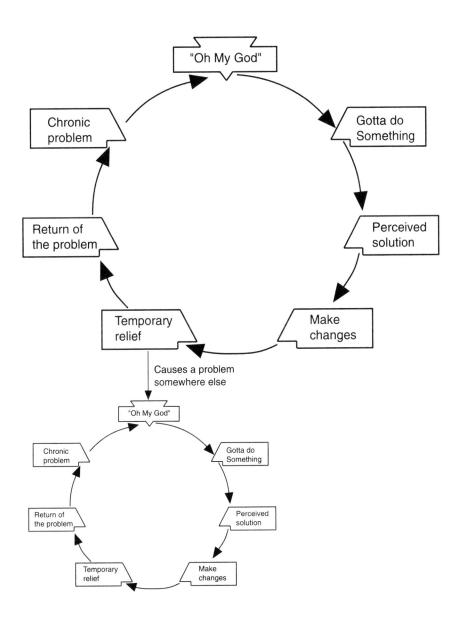

Figure 2–2 Typical Problem Solving

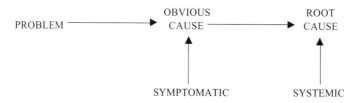

Figure 2–3 Determining Root Cause

Flowchart

This concept addresses the issue of clearly identifying the flow of each process in the agency. There are approximately 14 distinct functions or processes in the average home care agency:

1. inquiry/intake process
2. insurance/credit verification process
3. data entry process
4. scheduling process
5. service delivery process
6. quality assurance/utilization review process
7. medical records process
8. personnel/recruiting process
9. staff development process
10. payroll process
11. billing process
12. collection process
13. accounts payable/supplies process
14. sales/marketing process

Each of these functions should have a flowchart that delineates the flow of tasks, identifies where decision points are, and identifies alternative courses of action based on a positive or negative response to the decision.

There is nothing new or particularly statistical about the flowchart. However, the flowchart ensures that everyone agrees on how the process works. Without this agreement, variation will become rampant. A sample flowchart is provided in Figure 2–4.

There are different levels of flowcharting. The person or group completing the flowchart should determine the desired level based on their needs:

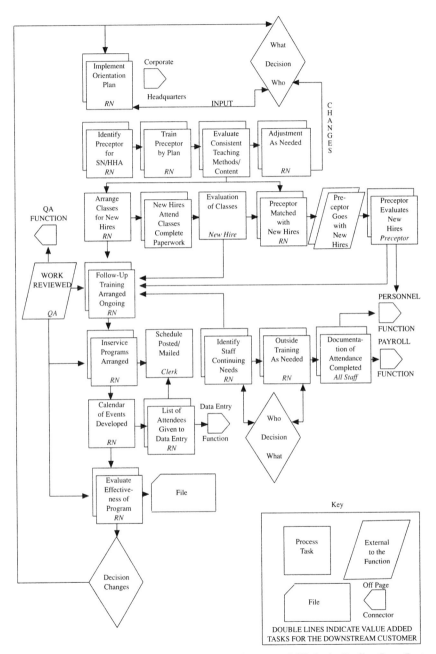

Figure 2-4 Staff Development Process. *Source:* Courtesy of Kimberly Quality Care, Boston, Massachusetts.

Level 0. A macro view of the agency. This view will encompass each of the 14 major processes that make up the organization. This is the high-level view from 10,000 feet above the ground.

Level 1. A micro view of the agency that "blows up" each of the major (14) functions to show each task associated with the process. This chart will take one of the processes from the Level 0 chart and detail it from 1,000 feet above the ground. For example, one of the processes from the Level 0 chart will be staff development. The Level 1 chart for this process will detail all the tasks associated with staff development, including how and when to fill out forms. An example of a Level 1 flowchart is illustrated in Figure 2–4.

Level 2. This is a mini-micro view at ground level encompassing the data elements within each task. This level follows the blowup of a process, to the blowup of tasks, to the blowup of data elements required in each task. As in the example of staff development, the Level 2 flowchart will detail all the data elements required for each Level 1 task when a form or document is in use. Generally, Level 2 flowcharting is used for the development of computer systems as it lends itself to data mapping. It is, however, too detailed for general use in improvement opportunities. There are exceptions to every rule. The exception here is when the agency's improvement opportunity is to reduce paperwork for the nurses. In this case, Level 2 flowcharting is essential to identify all the necessary data elements and how many times they are written and the number of forms on which they are written.

The separation of levels in flowcharting helps the user to focus on what is important for the task at hand. There is no need to complicate an improvement process with hundreds of flowcharts. Use the level of flowchart most appropriate for the task.

Just as there are different levels of flowcharting, there are also different types of flowcharts that can assist the user, depending on the task. Types of flowcharts are:

Process Flowcharts. A graphic depiction of a process within boundaries established by the input and ending with the output of that process. This illustration is seen vertically within the organization and generally defines areas of responsibility.

Events Flowcharts. A graphic depiction of an event that crosses process boundaries. The event starts when triggered and continues until a new event is triggered (an admission, for example). These charts are seen horizontally within an organization and have multiple people responsibilities assigned at different points. These charts are especially good for computer programmers who see events as data flows through an agency. This type of flowchart is difficult for use in training or in operational definitions, however, since areas of responsibility become confused.

For the purpose of this text, we will be using process flowcharts at Level 1.

Team Interaction

Obtaining agreement on the flowchart or anything else requires teamwork. Teamwork is another cornerstone of quality improvement. Teams should be empowered to be responsible for improving processes. Before employees are placed on teams and expected to act as a synergistic unit, they must be trained in team dynamics. There are a number of excellent books on this subject and many training programs are commercially available. Therefore, it is not necessary to go into detail on this subject. However, for purposes of this text, there are some fundamentals to bear in mind:

- Teams should be chosen with great care to ensure that all members can contribute equally to the team mission.
- Teams should be given training either before or during an assignment in quality improvement. Minimally, training should cover team dynamics and quality tools and techniques.
- Teams should have a clearly articulated purpose with a beginning and ending time frame.
- Teams should spell out their areas of authority. There is nothing more disturbing to a team that has worked hard than a senior level person overturning or changing their work.
- Teams should have time made available during working hours to accomplish their objectives.
- Teams should have a leader to coordinate activities and communication.

The people who make up the teams for each of the processes to be improved should include those with the most intimate knowledge of the process—in other words, those who work in the process. The team should also include an upstream and downstream customer (discussed under Concept 3).

After the team for each process has been chosen, team members should be empowered to complete the job of designing or redesigning the operating system through the development of all the flowcharts needed.

When agreement is reached on how the process or function is currently flowing, the team should begin to make necessary changes in accordance with customer requirements. The first time a team sees the actual flow, members will recognize steps that are redundant or without value. These can be deleted easily. The rule of thumb to use in the design of a process is that for every input from the upstream customer, the function or process should add value before passing it to the downstream customer. If no value is added, the task should be reconsidered.

Special attention should also be paid to tasks done for security reasons. For example, a billing clerk may review the UB–82 (the uniform billing form used nationally); the quality assurance nurse may review the UB–82; the office manager may review the UB–82; and the branch manager may review the UB–82. Each person reviews to make sure everything is right. It is easily seen that this duplication wastes valuable resources and delays billing. All of these people believe they must do their own review to ensure accuracy. The need for this level of security addresses a process problem that can be remedied through building quality into the process rather than trying to inspect in quality at the back end.

The following are some simple steps that will ensure good technique in flowcharting processes:

1. Establish process boundaries (where did the input [starting point] come from?).
2. Establish the ending point (what is the output and where will it go?).
3. Identify all necessary steps within the boundaries to transform the input into the output in sequential order.
4. Identify all decision points and alternative courses of action.
5. Eliminate tasks that add no value to the downstream customer.

After the team has agreed on how the flowchart looks, go through a final exercise designed to identify problem areas. A series of questions can be asked to assist the team to identify areas that require additional improvement:

1. Where are the problems occurring for this process?
2. What are the complaints?
3. Where do errors occur?
4. Are there any bottlenecks in the flow?
5. Is there agreement on all work methods and sequencing?
6. Does each task add value to the customer, or simply cost?
7. Has all backtracking been eliminated?

Operational Definition

After the team makes all the necessary adjustments to the process, it should be empowered to write operational definitions for the new process. This is a tedious responsibility, but one that will ultimately determine the success of the operation. Operational definition gives meaning to concepts and sets the parameters within which people are empowered to operate and make decisions. Operational definitions should be specific and quantifiable. Remember the blue shirt example? The reason people gave different answers on how many blue shirts were in the audience was because the requirements were not specific enough to form an operational definition of exactly what to do. In this example, there was no operational definition of the word blue. Reasonable people will differ on meaning; there was also no specific definition of shirt (do blouses count?) If the instructions were refined to count all the men's navy blue shirts, it is more likely that the numbers would be the same.

The principles for clarity in definition are the same for processes as they are for audits or anything else. That is, parameters should be established within which decisions can be made. Needless to say, all operational definitions should be committed to paper and circulated to the appropriate staff.

Concept 3

> Every process in health care has an upstream and downstream customer who will determine quality at the point of interaction.

The process or function under study should be considered in extended terms.[4] For example, before a process can begin, something has to happen to initiate the function. As in the case of staff development (see Figure 2–4), the upstream customer is corporate headquarters, which provides the overall orientation plan. In other words, the local office cannot begin to implement the plan until corporate headquarters gives them the plan. In this case, headquarters is the upstream customer. Additionally, QA is also an upstream customer, since the input provided becomes the basis for future programming.

The downstream customer is the one who becomes the immediate or direct recipient of the output from the process. Staff development has several downstream customers: employees, the personnel function, the data entry function, and the payroll function. The end user, or patient, is farther downstream from this process, except in the case of the preceptor and new hire interacting on the first visit. In this case, the patient has primary contact with the preceptor and new hire and only indirect contact with staff development. Figure 2–5 illustrates this concept.

Customers can be either internal (employees) or external (patients, physicians). Requirements of both groups must be taken into consideration if quality is to be achieved. Knowing the customers of each process and their position relative to upstream or downstream will clarify the location of the points of interaction, and the types of interactions.

Quality is determined through points of interaction with customers. Earlier we discussed that quality in perception and quality in fact hold equal value. Under this CQI concept, quality in perception is called *relational quality* and will be

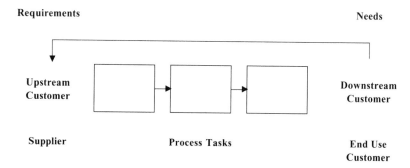

Figure 2–5 The Extended Process. *Source:* Gitlow, H., and Gitlow, S., *The Deming Guide to Quality and Competitive Position,* Prentice-Hall, 1987.

discussed in detail in Chapter 4. Relational quality is determined when a customer comes into contact with some aspect of the agency and forms an opinion. For example, if the nurse is drawing blood, the patient generally does not know if this procedure is technically correct. However, the patient will judge how the nurse treats him or her during the procedure. Was the nurse empathetic? Did he or she explain the procedure first? Was the patient put at ease? Did the nurse display a warm, friendly attitude? Did the nurse appear to know what to do? The answers to these questions will determine if the patient has a perception of quality based on the relationship formed or continued at the visit.

Everyone has met nurses that are highly competent yet appear cold. The thought may have occurred that if ever you were comatose, this is the nurse you would want. However, if you are alert, chances are you would want a warm, friendly nurse to care for you in sickness. A "cold" nurse may be technically competent, but most people would rather be cared for by a "warm" personality.

Quality is determined at the point of interaction and is dependent on human factors. These factors form an overall experience with the agency that will transcend the technical aspects of quality. For example, if the technical procedures during the course of treatment were perfect but the nurse was not friendly or did not respect the patient, the perception of quality would be poor. On the other hand, if the caregiving experience was good but the office incompetently handled the billing, the patient would still perceive a lack of quality.

While relational quality is based on human factors, there are some elements that form key characteristics and are universally applicable to all customers. These key elements are:

1. Convenience: Convenience is a concept that is only now becoming recognized in the health care industry. Convenience has always been part

of the attraction of home care; however, the issue of convenience is more prominent in CQI. Convenience means it is easy to do business with the agency and encompasses the entire relationship experience. It covers all aspects of relational quality including the caregiving experience, billing, communication, planning, and scheduling. Each interaction with the agency must be made convenient for the patient, not the agency. All too often patients are scheduled at the convenience of the caregiver rather than the other way around.

2. Consistency: Consistency in the delivery of home care is a major issue in CQI. Lack of consistency increases variation, which decreases quality performance. It is interesting to note that many customers would rather have lesser service rendered consistently than excellent service one time and undistinguished service another. Without consistency, planning becomes impossible. Agencies with multiple locations have an additional consistency challenge: ensuring that all offices provide the same level of quality services. Consistency of delivered services starts with the Deming model explained in Chapter 1.

3. Customization: The third quality element is customization. Home care agencies generally do a very good job in this aspect of quality. While customization in plans of treatment and other medical documentation is necessary when dealing with a diverse population, it is not the only source of potential customization. Most agency standards are to bill either once a week or monthly. Some patients may prefer to be billed at a different time.

    There must be a balance between customization and standardization. With standardization comes the ability to reduce variation and thereby improve quality. Standardization also provides the opportunity to decrease costs. Customization should be balanced against these features to allow for optimization of customer preference within predefined parameters.

4. Cycle-Time: Tom Peters, lecturer and management consultant, predicted that cycle-time will be the number one competitive advantage of the 1990s.[5] Consumers are demanding faster, cheaper, and better-than-ever services. Of these, faster is the most important. With today's fast-paced life styles, faster is not only definitely better, it is the only way to stay in business.

    With patients being discharged from hospitals sicker than ever before, waiting 24 hours to start care may no longer be appropriate. How long does it take your agency to provide therapy services? What happens when a caregiver calls in sick? Can a replacement be found immediately? How long does it take to complete the discharge summary? All these questions involve cycle-time that can be improved.

It should be noted that quality enables cycle-time reduction and cycle-time drives quality improvement. This concept is contrary to the old belief that a quality job took longer. CQI provides the methods by which quality becomes a more efficient means of achieving goals within smaller and smaller time frames. This becomes possible because of the reduction of waste, simplification of processes, and less rework from the ability to do it right the first time.

When looking at all the points of interaction where customers can form opinions about quality, the foregoing quality elements can guide decisions on process improvements. While improving processes, it becomes apparent that some of the so-called "back room" functions are really front-line customer contact positions and should be treated accordingly. Billing and collections are actually front-line customer contact positions, not back room functions. Personnel in these positions should, like the sales staff, receive customer service training.

To further define the extended process from a customer's perspective, it should be noted that the upstream customer becomes the supplier of input to the process and the downstream customer becomes the end user of the output from the process. Each of the subsequent tasks performed within the process should add value for the downstream customer. This is further illustrated in Figure 2–6.

Concepts 4–6

Concepts 4, 5, and 6 are all statistical in nature. These concepts form the foundation for some of the tools and techniques used in CQI. Because each of these concepts has statistics as their foundation, we will review them as a group.

Every process generates or produces output that can be either measured or counted.

Every process has a pattern or shape that is discernable when viewed in graphic form. This shape becomes the basis for all statistical studies and improvement efforts and is commonly referred to as the bell-shaped curve.

Every process will have variation. Variation is a natural state but is the enemy of quality.

These three concepts are the very heart of continuous quality improvement. They are the ones that will require the basic tools in statistical methods.

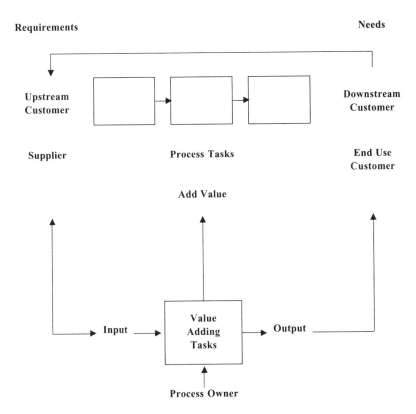

Figure 2–6 The Extended Process

Statistical Principles

Statistics play an important part in CQI. A review of some of the principles of statistics is helpful.

Descriptive Statistics. Statistics are used to describe and summarize data that are collected. When data are collected, they usually identify a subset of all the data possible. All of the possible observations are called the *population.* The subset of data is known as the *sample.*

There are two different types of data that can be observed and measured. *Variables* data are measurements. Examples include blood pressure and temperatures. *Attributes* data are characteristics that can be counted. Typically this is viewed as data that can be classified as good versus bad, or data that requires a choice between two answers. For example, in a utilization review (UR) context, the question may be, "Is the clinical note payable by the intermediary?" The "yes" answers go on to be billed, the "no" answers are referred to staff development or QA.

When the information collected is variables data there are several statistics that can be calculated.

Measures of Central Tendency. Central tendency shows the location of the data. While often simply referred to as the "average," there are three statistics commonly used as measures of central tendency.

The *arithmetic mean* is the average of the values. Generally shown with the symbol, $\bar{x}$, the arithmetic mean is calculated by finding the sum of all the values and then dividing by the number of values.

Example: Find the arithmetic average of the following data points:

$$8, 3, 6, 7, 9, 4, 5, 4, 8, 8, 4$$

The sum of the 11 numbers is 66. When this is divided by 11 (number of values) the arithmetic mean is 6.

The *median* is the middle value. In other words, there are an equal number of values on both sides of the median. The median is the point at which 50 percent of the numbers fall above and 50 percent fall below the center. The median is usually determined by placing the values in numerical order and identifying the value that is midway through the listing.

Example: Find the median of the following data points:

$$9, 2, 6, 7, 9, 4, 5, 4, 8, 8, 4$$

The first step is to put the 11 numbers in order, from smallest to largest.

$$2, 4, 4, 4, 5, 6, 7, 8, 8, 9, 9$$

Because there are 11 numbers, the median, or middle, value will be the sixth. In this example that is 6. In other words, there are five numbers on either side of six.

The *mode* is the most frequently occurring value in the sample.

Example: Find the mode of the following data points:

$$8, 2, 6, 7, 9, 4, 5, 4, 8, 9, 4$$

In this sample we have one "2", three "4s", one "5", one "6", one "7", two "8s" and two "9s". The most frequently occurring value is 4.

Measures of central tendency are used to identify where the data are centered. Once the center is known, it can be compared with where the data should be centered to evaluate how the data perform regarding the target location. The location refers to the values placement on a control chart or in reference to the bell-shaped curve.

Measures of Variability. Measures of variability show how widely dispersed the data are.

The *standard deviation* shows how the sample data are dispersed about the central location, or average. In other words, how wide is the variation in the data? While the calculation of this statistic is a bit complicated, the main use of the standard deviation is when data are interpreted.

The *range* is the difference between the largest and smallest value in a sample. Example: Find the range of the following data points:

$$8, 2, 6, 7, 9, 4, 5, 4, 8, 9, 4$$

The largest value is 9. The smallest value is 2. The difference is 9–2=7.

Shape. The shape of the distribution can provide very useful information about the sample and the population. If the sample is tabulated by frequency of occurrence, in a histogram, the shape of the histogram can tell much about the sample population.

The *normal distribution* is a bell-shaped curve (see Figure 2–7). It describes the way many data are usually (normally) distributed. This type of distribution is tall toward the center and tails off rapidly toward the edge of the distribution. When data are normally distributed we know the following about the variability of the data:

- Within 1 standard deviation in either direction of the process average we expect to find about 68 percent of all possible values or occurrences.
- Within 2 standard deviations in either direction of the process average we expect to find about 95.5 percent of all possible values or occurrences.
- Within 3 standard deviations in either direction of the process average we expect to find about 99.7 percent of all possible values or occurrences.

Central Limit Theorem. An important statistical relationship is expressed in what is called the central limit theorem. This theorem states that, when we take a large number of samples, no matter what the shape of the original distribution, the distribution of sample averages will always be normally distributed. When we couple that with the information about proportion of data within a specified number of standard deviations we can make some very accurate predictions about process performance.

Defect Location Diagram

The defect location diagram is one of the specific statistical tools that will turn CQI concepts into actionable issues.

This diagram is one that all in the health care industry will readily recognize. It is usually a model of the front and back of the body and is used to mark scarring, skin breakdown, or other anomalies. These diagrams are almost always found in

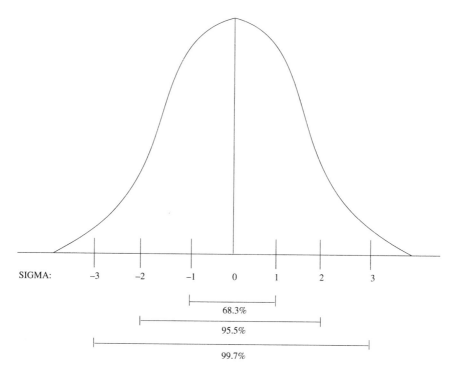

SIGMA: -3   -2   -1   0   1   2   3

68.3%

95.5%

99.7%

Figure 2-7 Normal Curve (Mean—0/Standard Deviations Marked). *Source:* Bliersbach, C.M., *Guide to Health Care Quality Management,* p. 20.10, National Association of Quality Assurance Professionals, 1990.

the history and physical portion of the admission paperwork, generally in the nursing assessment.

In this context, however, the defect location diagram takes on a broader meaning. Remember that the concept is to measure or count those things that are meaningful. The purpose, as stated throughout this book, is not only to solve the problem but to prevent it from recurring—hence, continuous improvement. The defect location diagram is an excellent tool to use in the risk management program for identifying locations of injury to the body. Over time, the risk manager may identify that 32 out of 40 employee injuries were injuries to the back. The defect location diagram will visually identify trends that would otherwise take detailed analysis to reveal.

Run Charts[6]

Because variation is a natural state, it is not possible to predict individual outcomes exactly. However, if a process or function is stable (meaning that there are no special causes), the pattern of variability is predictable. For example, in a run chart on total visits performed each month by a typical agency in Florida, the prediction is that the winter months will see an increase in visits over the summer months. A run chart is a visual depiction of trends in the agency. Run charts are usually trended over time and should be compared to the same period of time. Using the same example of total visits performed each month, the 1994 figures should be compared to 1993 and 1992.

The comparisons of like periods of time would not hold if the agency were in a growth mode and wanted to compare growth from month to month. An example of a run chart is found in Figure 2–8.

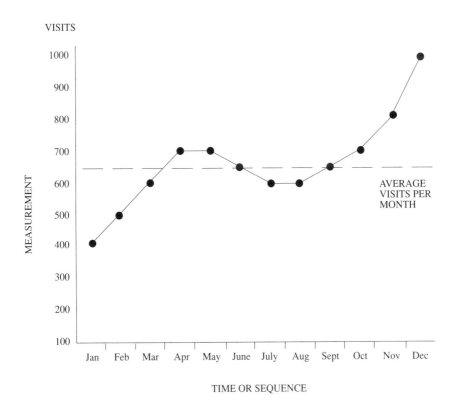

Figure 2–8 Run Chart

Histograms

The histogram allows the visual display of data in a form that shows the frequency of occurrence (frequency distribution) and pattern of distribution (bell-shaped curve).[7] It is used to display the distribution of data by bar graphing the number of units in each category. The histogram will visually display the amount of variation in any process and is, therefore, a very important tool. The histogram will look something like Figure 2–9.

Scatter Diagram

Scatter diagrams are used to determine whether two different variables are correlated or have a relationship. This tool is used to see whether there is a positive or negative effect relationship between the variables, e.g., the more the plotted points go in a straight line, the tighter the relationship.[8] If the line is upward in movement, the relationship is said to be positive. If the line is downward, it is a negative correlation.

Numerous regression analysis computer programs are available today that provide more complexity than the correlation of only two variables. These

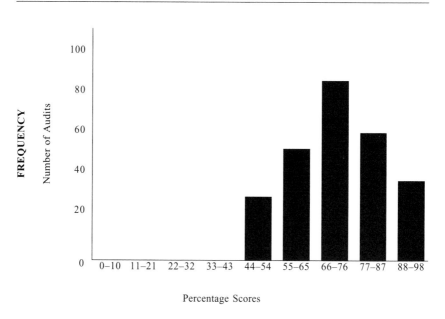

Percentage Scores

DISTRIBUTION

Figure 2–9 Histogram

programs can show correlations between numerous variables and should be considered if the agency wants to do detailed analysis in this area. These computerized tools are excellent for analysis of customer satisfaction results. An example of a scatter diagram is illustrated in Figure 2–10.

Variation

Variation is present in every process that is measured. There are two distinct types of variation. *Normal variation* is the variation always present in each process. It is due to many random causes, such as training variability, measurement system variability, and environmental variability. This type of variation results from the normal workings of the process and is management controllable. Deming attributes 94 percent of problems in process outcomes to this type of variation and calls it "common cause" variation. *Abnormal variation* is present

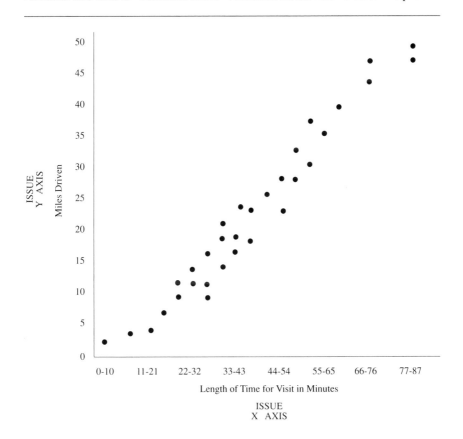

Figure 2–10 Scatter Diagram

when special or assignable causes are present. Deming defined abnormal variation as special causes, which he said account for approximately 6 percent of the problems from process outcomes. These special causes are attributable to a specific person, technique, or other assignable source. Examples of abnormal variation causes include equipment that breaks or an unskilled person performing a technical procedure.

Control Charts

The control chart is one of the most important tools for CQI. The control chart shows the variability of the process characteristic being measured as time passes. The control chart shows the limits of expected normal variation. The control chart differentiates between normal and abnormal variation or special and common cause variations.

Control limits show the expected range of normal variation. These are usually calculated using three standard deviation (sigma) limits from the average. This implies that 99.7 percent of the occurrences will fall between the upper and lower control limits (see Figure 2–7). When a process is in control it means that only normal variation is present. When a process is in control it does not mean that the process is behaving in an acceptable manner. It only means that the process is performing in a "normal" way given its procedures. In order to improve a process in control, management will have to change the procedures governing the operation of the process. A process in control has predictive abilities. In other words, a process that is in a state of statistical control will continue to perform within the three sigma control limits until the process is changed. When a process is out of control it means that abnormal variation is present. When a process is out of control it does not mean that the process is behaving in an unacceptable manner. A process that is out of control indicates that a special cause is present and should be removed. As long as special or abnormal variation is present, the process has no predictive value. Before an out-of-control process can be improved, all special causes must be removed. The process must be brought into a state of statistical control before improvements can have a reliable effect.

As previously stated, Deming believes that over 94 percent of all problems with processes are common cause occurrences or normal variation and that the remaining 6 percent are special causes or abnormal variation.

The responsibility for change to improve quality rests either with management or with an individual, depending on the problem or opportunity. Accordingly, Deming delineated two means of process improvement: changing the common causes that are systematic and removing the special causes that produce nonrandom variation within the process (or procedure). Common causes can include lack of sufficient staff development, poor procedural definition, lack of adequate supplies and equipment, etc. Special causes can include lack of a specific skill, a new employee, etc.

Deming said that common causes are the responsibility of management to resolve while special causes must be resolved by the individual employee. A closer look at this issue requires a control chart. Control limits are statistically defined and plotted on a control chart. Any data points outside the control limits indicate that the process that produced the data is out of control. This means that the process is not reliable, or, in other words, that the process is not predictive of future performance. Out-of-control processes also indicate that there is wide variation in the outcome from the process, which indicates poor quality.

Common causes of problems have to do with policy, procedure, systems, or other issues that affect a wide variety of outcomes. Special causes, on the other hand, are a result of individual action. It is logical to assume that if special causes make up only 6 percent of the problems, then our efforts should be concentrated on solving the common causes of problems.

The best way to identify processes out of control is to do a control chart. The method of control charting is defined as statistical process control (SPC). The form was developed by Walter A. Shewhart while at Bell Labs in the 1930s and later refined by Deming in a well known paper, "On Statistical Theory of Errors." The paper delineated random variation from variation that could indicate special causes.

Deming further argued that until a process was in a state of statistical control, no real improvements could be made that would have a sustained effect. Since processes in control had predictive outcomes, Deming believed quality could be improved with sustained results. He also believed that productivity would be improved with controlled processes. Quality and productivity were not to be traded off against each other as generally believed. Deming has proven that productivity is a by-product of quality and of doing things right the first time.[9]

Because management was responsible, in Deming's view, for 94 percent of quality problems, management had to take the lead in changing the systems and processes that created those problems. For example, consistent quality of incoming supplies could not be expected where buyers were told to shop for price, or were not given the tools for assessing a supplier's quality. Management had to take the lead in developing long-term relationships with vendors, working with vendors to improve and maintain quality, training its own purchasing department in statistical quality control, requiring statistical evidence of quality from vendors, and insisting that specifications be complete. Only when management had changed purchasing systems and procedures could buyers be expected and able to do their job in a new way. Once top management was seriously committed to quality, lower-level personnel would be more likely to take action on problems that were within their control.[10]

Probability rules could determine whether variation was random, i.e., whether it was due to chance. Random variation occurs within statistically determined limits and should be plotted on the control chart. If variation remained within those limits, the process was a stable one, and said to be in control. As long as nothing changed the process, future variation could be easily predicted, for it would remain indefinitely within the same statistical limits.

Data of this sort should be normally collected and plotted on control charts kept by the employees themselves. Such charts graphically plot actual performance readings and depict the upper and lower control limits for that characteristic, which were statistically determined (see Figure 2–11).

Once a process was in control, readings that fell outside the limits indicated a special cause. When the cause of such nonrandom variation was found and removed, the system returned to its stable state. Deming warns:

> Courses in statistics often commence with the study of distribution and comparison of distributions. Students are not warned in classes nor in books that for analytic purposes (such as to improve a process), distributions and calculations of mean, mode . . . and standard deviation serve no useful purpose for improvement of a process *unless the data were produced in state of statistical control.* The first step in the examination of data is, accordingly, to question the state of statistical control that produced the data. The easiest way to examine data is plot points in order of occurrence to learn whether any use can be made of the distribution of the data.[11]

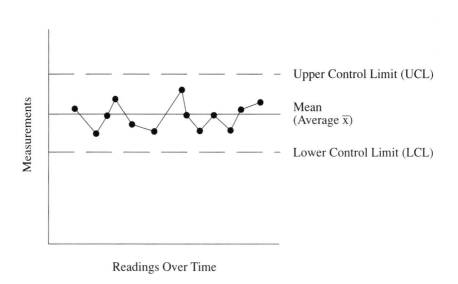

Figure 2–11 A Typical Control Chart

In simpler terms, Deming is stating that one cannot use data to predict future actions or occurrences unless that data were produced by a system in control. The best way to determine whether the system is in control is to do a control chart. All situations resulting in points outside the upper or lower control limits must be remedied before a state of statistical control will occur.

Types of Control Charts

There are two types of control charts that are commonly used. These are the variables charts and the attributes charts. The most commonly used variables chart is the $\bar{x}$ (bar) and R chart. The proportion defective is a frequently used attributes chart. An example of this use in home care would be to calculate the proportion of "good" plan of treatments (POTs) versus those that had an error. The attributes chart can be used for this purpose. If all the points fall within the control limits, it would indicate that management would need to change the process if improvements are to be made.

$\bar{X}$ *Bar and R Chart (variables).* This chart examines the performance of sample averages and sample ranges. The averages are selected because they will, in the long run, always be normally distributed. The ranges show the variability of the process. Since Dr. Deming stresses that CQI involves reducing process variability, this is an important characteristic to chart. This chart is especially helpful when data are not normally distributed. Using averaging for large populations of numbers will automatically distribute the data in the normal pattern. Like predictive value for processes in a state of statistical control, normal distribution must occur before certain statistical methods can be applied with any degree of accuracy.

Control limit calculations are shown in Exhibit 2–3 and a table of factors appears in Table 2–1. These limits show us the expected range of normal variability.

Attributes Charts. Attributes charts also show the expected range of normal variability for attributes that are counted for a process. Most typically, the proportion or percentage of errors is the characteristic that is charted.

The proportion defective chart is called a p chart. P will indicate the process capability for the calculations of good or bad. The p chart will indicate what proportion of bad or rejects exist in the entire population. The concepts used here are extremely important to home care providers who monitor the issue of statistical sampling as a basis for intermediary denials. While the issue of sampling will not be discussed in this context, the application of the findings is conceptually the same. Let us use the example of the clinical note. Upon review, a decision is rendered that the note is payable or not. Those deemed not payable will be classified as rejects. The formula follows:

Exhibit 2–3 Formulas for Calculating Control Limits for $\overline{X}$ and R Chart

---

Calculate the average ($\overline{X}$) and range (R) of each subgroup:

$$\overline{X} = \frac{X1 + X2 + X3 \ldots}{n \text{ (number in sample)}}$$

$$R = Xmax - Xmin$$

Calculate the average range ($\overline{R}$) and the process average ($\overline{\overline{X}}$):

$$\overline{\overline{X}} = \frac{\overline{X}1 + \overline{X}2 + \overline{X}3 \ldots}{k \text{ (number of subgroups)}}$$

$$\overline{R} = \frac{R1 + R2 + R3 \ldots}{k \text{ (number of subgroups)}}$$

Calculate the control limits:

$$\text{UCL}\,\overline{x} = \overline{\overline{X}} + A_2 \times \overline{R} \qquad \text{LCL}\,\overline{x} = \overline{\overline{X}} - A_2 \times \overline{R}$$
$$\text{UCL R} = D_4 \times \overline{R} \qquad\qquad \text{LCL R} = D_3 \times \overline{R}$$

Plot the chart on standard graph paper.
Refer to Table 2–1 for the factors needed for A_2 and D_3 & D_4.

Source: Reprinted from *The Memory Jogger,* pp. 53–54, © Copyright 1988, GOAL/QPC, 13 Branch Street, Methuen, MA, 01844. Tele. 508-685-3900. Used with permission.

$$p = \frac{\text{number of rejects in subgroup}}{\text{number inspected in subgroup}}$$

$$\overline{p} = \frac{\text{total number of rejects}}{\text{total number inspected}}$$

$$\text{UCL } p = \overline{p} + \frac{3\sqrt{\overline{p}\,(1 - \overline{p})}}{\sqrt{n}} \qquad \text{LCL } p = \overline{p} - \frac{3\sqrt{\overline{p}\,(1 - \overline{p})}}{\sqrt{n}}$$

Most of the work home care agencies have done for quality improvement use attributes data. When using this type of data, the output measures will generally follow a bimodal distribution. In other words, the distribution using the histogram will reveal what appears to be two dominant peaks. (See Figure 2–12.) This is to be expected since there are only two choices in this scenario.

Table 2–1 Factors for $\overline{X}$ and R Charts

NUMBER OF OBSERVATIONS IN SUBGROUP (n)	FACTORS FOR X CHART A_2	FACTORS FOR R CHART LOWER D_3	UPPER D_4
2	1.880	0	3.268
3	1.023	0	2.574
4	0.729	0	2.282
5	0.577	0	2.114
6	0.483	0	2.004
7	0.419	0.076	1.924
8	0.373	0.136	1.864
9	0.337	0.184	1.816
10	0.308	0.223	1.777

Source: Reprinted from *The Memory Jogger*, pp. 53–54, © Copyright 1988, GOAL/QPC, 13 Branch Street, Methuen, MA 01844. Telephone: 508-685-3900. Used with permission.

The p chart is used to determine whether the number or proportion of "bad, no, late, unfilled," etc. is stable over time. It should be pointed out that attributes charts are no substitute for the variables chart. The attributes charts have no power to predict impending trouble if the process is not producing any rejects. They are, however, very useful to tell us the average proportion of nonconformance and to alert us to changes in that proportion. Additionally, the attributes charts can help us discover out-of-control high or low changes in the proportion and subsequently to find special causes. These charts can also suggest places where variables charts will prove useful for diagnosing quality problems.[12]

Specification Limits

Control limits are statistically calculated and show the expected normal process variability when the process is stable. The stability of the process is necessary to predict its future performance. Without stability, no prediction can be valid. Control limits, however, do not address whether or not a process is behaving in an acceptable fashion.

Control limits have become known as the "voice of the process" in that they indicate the amount of variation found within the process given the current state. On the other hand, specification limits address the performance of the process. Specification limits are representative of customer expectations and customer requirements. *Process characteristics must be within specification limits for the process to be acceptable to the customer.* In other words, specification limits are considered the "voice of the customer."

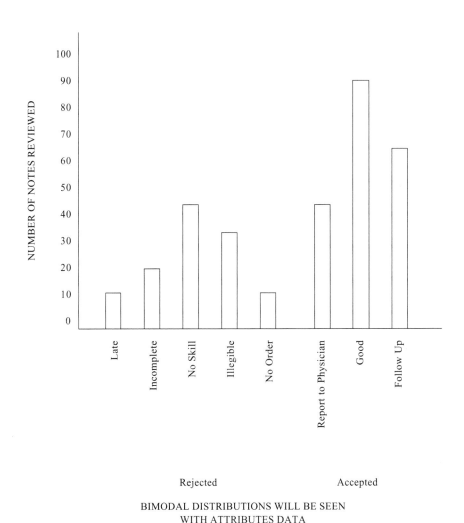

Figure 2–12 Bimodal Distribution

While health care providers are adept at working with spec limits, they are not accustomed to working with control limits. The entire underlying meaning to the issue of continuous quality improvement is that consistently meeting the needs of customers will not happen until all of the processes that support the service delivery system are stable and in control. This will necessitate the understanding and use of control charts by anyone responsible for process.

Concept 7

> Every process has key quality characteristics that add value for the
> downstream customer upon which standards can be set.

Key quality characteristics are the most important attributes of customer
service determined from customer-based research. Generally, the key quality
characteristics are reliability, responsiveness, assurance of quality, empathy,
and intangibles such as reputation and community image. The key quality characteristics will become the service features around which standards should be set.
Once standards are set, a measurement system must be developed to measure the
agency's performance against the key characteristics. The measurement system
data should focus on two areas: (1) the most important attributes of customer
service, and (2) the attributes that serve to protect the agency's interests.

The concept of standards for key quality characteristics presents a difficult
shift in thinking for most agency personnel who have been trained to believe that
standards are those imposed by the Health Care Financing Administration
(HCFA) or the Joint Commission. While these standards certainly are important,
HCFA's criteria is based on a minimum level of overall performance and is
focused on protecting the government's interest in the delivery of home care to
Medicare beneficiaries. The Joint Commission, on the other hand, sets guidelines
that, if followed, ensure the agency can perform quality services, by the Joint
Commission's definition.

No standards of performance under either organization look at key quality
characteristics from the patient's perspective. Previously, we discussed the
concept of external and internal customers. For the measurement system to be
effective, the agency must have standards that serve both groups. Patients, as
external customers, need standards that ensure the desired behaviors. Internal
customers need standards that reduce errors and failure costs.

For example, a key quality characteristic may be the reliability of the nurse
coming to the home at a mutually agreed time. The standard of performance may
be 95 percent on time visits. It will not help to improve the agency's performance
unless these standards are tracked and reported. Employees must perceive that
the key quality characteristics are important to management. If management
never looks at or addresses performance standards, they will not be important to
the staff.

One of the best ways to demonstrate the importance of performance standards
is to link them to the employee appraisal system for compensation and/or bonus.
These standards should also be linked to any reward and recognition system the
agency has. This aligns the customer's requirements to conformance of those
requirements to the compensation system. This alignment is crucial for the

overall success of a quality system. All too often, agency administrators stress quality, but reward for profitability. This disconnect between what is said and what is done created the phrase, "walk-the-talk," which is discussed in more detail in Chapter 3.

The number of standards is another important issue that agency administrators must address. The Joint Commission has over 500 standards for the delivery of home care. HCFA has the Federal Conditions of Participation. There is no way an administrator can place importance on all of these standards and do any of them well. There are two approaches to this dilemma. The first is to empower staff to be accountable for standards of performance within their scope of responsibility. It is recommended that no more than three standards be imposed on any one person. Standards should be imposed on the person responsible for the behavior, not the supervisor. Supervisory personnel should be accountable for the overall performance of the department.

Some confusion seems to exist over the issue of accountability as it relates to the team-building process. The two concepts are not mutually exclusive. Deming believes that if two people are responsible for the same thing, then no one is responsible for it. That is not to say that a team is not accountable for the entire process or department. It is to say that each team member is accountable for a specific component of the process and accountable for that component's standard. The team as a whole is accountable for the process as a whole. Like any good team, each component is better when combined with the others. The burden of standards can be distributed to each member of the team and each contributes equally to the success of the whole.

In the second approach, HCFA and Joint Commission standards should be considered a normal part of doing business and be completely documented in operational definition rather than standards of performance. This approach allows the agency to always be prepared for on-site visits by HCFA and the Joint Commission without the usual preparation time. With these standards as a normal part of operational definition, there is sufficient opportunity to gear performance standards to the users of home care services.

The following is a general guide on the establishment of key quality characteristics:

- Standards of quality should be jointly defined by the upstream and downstream customer.
- The standards should be directly related to meeting all customers' needs but are driven by the downstream customer.
- The standards should be a part of a regular systematic feedback system incorporating objective, quantifiable data.
- Quality characteristics should be limited in scope to the important few.

- All standards should be viewed statistically over time.
- The standards will change as they are met consistently. (They will be increased.)

Some additional tools are available to assist the teams in developing the quality characteristics and standards of performance. The following tools can also be used for any other problem-solving situation.

Brainstorming

Brainstorming is used to solicit a large number of ideas on a specific problem or opportunity for improvement. Brainstorming provides a free-thinking, non-threatening, creative environment without judgment or repercussions.

Every team member sits silently for about five minutes and writes all of his or her ideas on paper. One team member is chosen to record exactly what is said by each person. Each person reads one issue at a time from his or her list. There can be no censorship or interruptions from any other member. Team members may piggyback off other ideas. All members may pass when they choose. The session is over when each team member passes consecutively.

When the idea gathering ends, discussion may begin. During this phase, ideas may be grouped together and otherwise modified for clarity. Once the discussion winds down, each team member should vote on each issue using a simple 1, 3, or 5 vote plan. For example, very important issues are given a 5, and so on. Each team member can spend up to a maximum of 30 votes.

The vote counts are for the purpose of forcing each team member to prioritize the issues he or she thinks are important and limit the boundaries of actionable items.

It is very important that the rules be followed as they were developed to allow for maximum creativity.

Pareto Chart

Vilfredo Pareto was a nineteenth-century economist who developed the Pareto Principle based on his studies of the distribution of wealth. Pareto found that 80 percent of his country's wealth was held by only 20 percent of the population. This maldistribution has held true for other studies and was generalized into statistical thinking by Joseph Juran. The 80/20 rule, as it has become known, distinguishes the "vital few" from the "trivial many." An illustration of the principle can be found in Figure 2–13.

The ideas that emerge from a brainstorming session can be put on a Pareto chart in order of the votes each idea receives. The team members will be able to quickly see which ideas have priority.

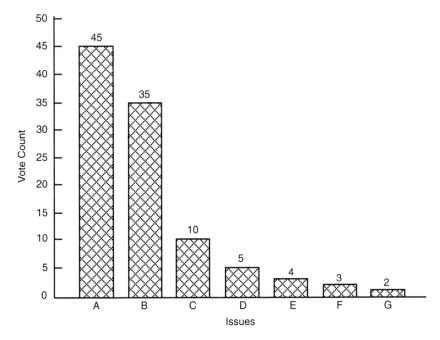

Figure 2–13 Pareto Chart. *Source:* Bliersbach, C.M., *Guide to Health Care Quality Management,* pp. 7–13, National Association of Quality Assurance Professionals, 1990.

Cause and Effect (Fishbone) Diagram

The fishbone diagram was developed by Kaoru Ishikawa. However, it was Walter Shewhart's[13] work on the definition of potential causes that propelled the wide use of the fishbone diagram in the quality improvement arena.

The effect is the desired outcome, and the causes are the "spine bones." Shewhart believed that all potential causes could be attributable to one of five categories:

1. Materials: Forms, supplies, information, etc.
2. Methods: Policy, procedure, practice, systems, etc.
3. Machines: Computers, blood pressure cuffs, etc.
4. People: Skill level, education, etc. (*Note:* The issues of orientation and training are considered a methods cause.)
5. Measurement system: What is being measured and how.

Figure 2–14 illustrates the Shewhart concept of the fishbone diagram form.

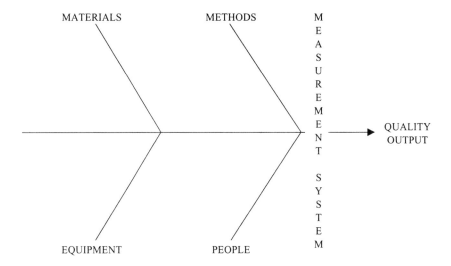

Figure 2–14 Fishbone Diagram. *Source:* Ishikawa, K., *Guide to Quality Control,* Asian Productivity Organization, Quality Resources, White Plains, New York, 1982.

The cause and effect diagram offers an excellent opportunity to categorize all the issues from the Pareto chart or directly from the brainstorming session. The grouping of problem issues by each category further assists the team in making work assignments for resolution. This diagram also helps the team to identify exactly what actions are necessary to correct the problem or improve a system or process.

Each of the tools for continuous quality improvement will assist the agency in its efforts toward total quality management. The key to success of the quality movement is to completely understand the difference between common cause and special cause variation. Causes that are attributable to management and those that are attributable to an individual employee will be seen only through statistical process control. Once they are identified, the resolutions can begin through brainstorming, Pareto charts, and fishbone diagrams. The purpose of these latter tools is to assist the agency in the identification of the root cause of the problem. Until this root cause is fully understood and remedied, the problem cannot be prevented.

Concept 8

Functions which do not add value for the downstream customer add waste cost to the corporation.

Waste Costs

Quality gurus have said that the customers' needs must be met at a price they are willing to pay. Those in home care administration know that all costs are included in the cost per visit. Indirect costs (administrative and general) offer the greatest opportunity to reduce costs. Deming said that between 40 to 60 percent of today's cost of administrative personnel and discrete functions are a direct result of not doing it right the first time.[14] For this reason, there is enormous opportunity for improved profitability and efficiency when systems are in place to prevent waste costs.

Deming defines waste cost in three categories:[15]

1. Costs that are attributable to the traditional inspection system. These costs are for inspection, review, and verification functions that would not be necessary if "we did it right the first time."
2. Cost of internal failure, e.g., mistakes that are caught and corrected before they leave the office.
3. Cost of external failure, e.g., mistakes that get to the downstream customer, which lead to expensive investigations, adjustments, penalties, and lawsuits.

These costs are invisible and not managed as well as they should be. As systems begin to improve using the tools of CQI, waste cost categories are replaced with the positive investments in prevention, analysis, and systematic control of quality.

It has been said that in the health care environment all occurrences warrant investigation. However, in the real world of highest value for the lowest dollar, resources must be allocated on a cause and effect basis. Therefore, only those takes that add value to the downstream customer should continue. All other tasks should be deleted. Value analysis is an excellent tool to objectively determine which tasks to delete. While this is a more advanced quality tool, the basics can be adapted for beginners. Steps in this process are:

1. Complete a process flowchart at Level 1 and number each task.
2. Identify the customers of the process and the relative position each holds, e.g., end user, indirect user, or supervisor. (These are generally seen as primary, secondary, and auxiliary customer positions.)
3. Using a team, identify which tasks have written specifications, regulations, or policies governing its existence.
4. Have the team identify any unarticulated expectations customers may have of this task.

5. Ask the team to identify any added value tasks in the flowchart. For purposes of this exercise, added value cannot be anything that has already been identified in either step 3 or 4.
6. Identify any task that intersects with a customer.
7. Analyze the results and delete no- or low-value tasks from the process. This is best accomplished using a matrix format.

This analytical process is necessary because most tasks that make up the process have evolved from some internal need in the agency. Because of this, those working on the task will feel a strong ownership about everything they do. It is painful to realize that some of the work done in the past has no present value to the customers.

While Deming skillfully articulated waste cost categories, we may want to look at these a little differently to include the customer perspective. The Deming categories, synopsized, are as follows:

- cost of typical inspection
- cost of internal duplication or inner security measures
- cost of external error or deficiency

There is another category of waste cost that cannot be quantified except by perception of the customer. Deming calls these costs unknowing and unknowable. These intangible costs are extracted from customers during the course of doing business and are in addition to the cost (price) of the service:

- complicated interactions with the agency
- burdens on the customers
- repeating information or steps
- wait time

Each cost in this waste category makes it more difficult to do business with the agency. As previously discussed, convenience or ease of doing business is one of the four quality elements. Agencies should examine their operating methods and eliminate any waste cost problems or complications to customers.

The tools identified in this chapter can be used in a variety of ways and should be taught to the agency's quality improvement teams. A basic understanding of the concepts outlined herein will help the reader apply CQI methods to improving patient care outcomes while reducing the overall cost of doing business for the agency and the customer.

It should now be apparent that customers, during the course of interaction with the agency, determine quality. While quality in fact (or, technical quality) has been the sole determinant of quality in the past, under CQI, it must share equally with relational quality. This book will attempt to apply tools to the improvement activities of both aspects of quality.

NOTES

1. U.S. General Accounting Office, *Management Practices, U.S. Companies Improve Performance through Quality Efforts* (Washington, D.C.: GAO/NSIAD-91-90).

2. B. Stralton, The Value of Implementing Quality, *Quality Progress,* vol. 24, no. 7 (The American Society of Quality Control, July, 1991), 70.

3. P.B. Crosby, *Quality Is Free* (New York: McGraw-Hill Publishing Co., 1979).

4. Excerpted from a speech given by Jim Tisdel, PhD, entitled, *The Development of a Company-Wide Quality and Productivity Improvement Process* (Qualpro Seminar, 1990).

5. TPG Communications, "Get Fast or Go Broke," with Tom Peters (video).

6. *Memory Jogger, A Pocket Guide of Tools for Continuous Quality Improvement* (Methuen, Mass.: GOAL/QPC, 1988).

7. Ibid.

8. Ibid.

9. W.E. Deming, *Out of Crisis* (Cambridge, Mass.: Massachusetts Institute of Technology, 1982).

10. *Notes on Quality—Views of Deming, Juran and Crosby, Garvin and March* (Boston, Mass.: HBS Case Studies, Harvard Business School, 1987, #687011).

11. Ibid.

12. Tisdel, *The Development of a Company-Wide Quality and Productivity Improvement Process.*

13. Statistical method from *The Viewpoint of Quality Control,* Walter A. Shewhart, 1939, Foreword by W. Edwards Deming, © 1986, p. i.

14. Deming, *Out of Crisis.*

15. Ibid.

Chapter 3

Total Quality Management

THE SINGLE FOCUS

The concepts of continuous quality improvement (CQI) have begun to take root and flourish in the field of home health. We in the home health care industry are beginning to feel more comfortable with these new concepts, and the fear of new tools is beginning to wear off.

A new language has been introduced and we are struggling to learn it. This new language speaks with a different voice—that of our customers.

We have redefined the old, introduced the new, and borrowed from our friends in manufacturing. All this we have done because we have an obligation to our patients and our employees. That obligation goes beyond service delivery and the receipt of a paycheck. It is the obligation of one friend to another to do everything possible to improve the quality of life we share.

Total quality management (TQM) is not a program; it is not even a concept. TQM is a way of life. TQM takes the principles and concepts of continuous quality improvement and applies them to everything we do, everything we say, and everything we are about. Those who believe in total quality management are the opposite of those who believe, "If it ain't broke, don't fix it."

TQM is about pulling together the entire agency into one focus, that of meeting the needs of the customer. It is about making decisions based on data to improve the effect downstream. It is about prevention.

TQM is becoming quality driven, customer focused, and value centered. Its structure is like a spiral instead of the traditional pyramid and works the same way. (See Figure 3–1.) Everyone in the agency is interdependent on everyone else. Everyone is focused and everything fits together. It's a team and it works.

Many home health providers use CQI interchangeably with TQM. These two concepts are similar in that they seek the same goals of improvement. They do,

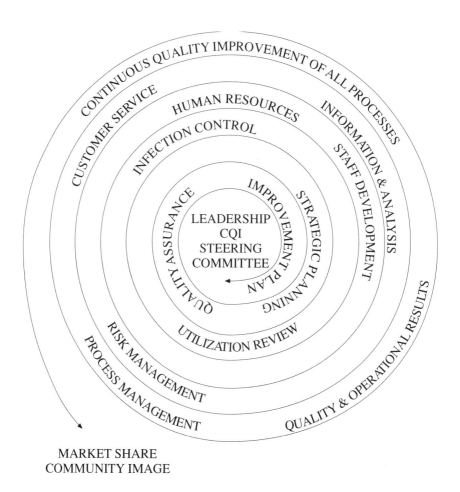

Figure 3–1 Total Quality Management

however, differ. As you will recall, CQI means continuous improvements in processes and requirements to better meet customer's expectations. TQM on the other hand, is about alignment. It is about integrity; consistently doing what you say you will do, and doing it right—the first time. TQM is mission based and value centered. TQM, therefore, is the effective management of technical, administrative, and human factors so as to achieve, sustain, and continually improve the agency's ability to meet customers' stated or implied needs.

The TQM system must be in alignment with the agency's mission. This alignment is critical to the success of any quality improvement initiative. There are three methods to assure alignment: (1) policy, (2) education, and (3) example.

Policy

The agency should state as its quality policy the intentions of management. The quality policy should be consistent with all other policies of the agency. The following is an example of a quality policy:

> The quality of all services shall be under control and all quality-related activities will be directed toward the reduction, elimination, and most importantly, the prevention of quality deficiencies.

> The objective of this quality policy is to achieve, sustain, and continually improve the agency's ability to meet the customer's stated or implied needs.

With this policy and objective statement, it will be easy to determine if there are any inconsistencies in other policies or procedures. Suppose the agency had another policy or procedures that read:

> Every UB–82 and its supporting documentation must be reviewed before being sent to the Intermediary.

This policy requires 100 percent back-end inspection, which increases the cost without determining control of the process that produced the claim forms. (There should be a p (control) chart to determine whether or not the process is in control. This control chart will also determine if management should change this process to improve the outcomes or if there is a special cause or abnormal variation.)

Additionally, the quality policy states that prevention will be the most important activity. Management philosophy must therefore change from defect detection to defect prevention. The policy requiring review of UB–82s has no support methodology for the prevention of errors nor is there a method to eliminate the recurrence of errors from future claims. The policy requiring review of UB–82s is, therefore, in conflict with the quality policy.

The articulation of a quality policy and removing inconsistencies from all other policies is a time-consuming task. However, it is critical if alignment is to occur. In the example presented, the policy on claim forms was a direct contradiction to the intentions of management toward quality. Allowing such contradictions will defeat the improvement initiatives because employees will not know what to do. In the absence of clear definitions, people will follow their own interpretation, which will increase variation in the process and cause quality to deteriorate.

Another consideration regarding policy is the system or processes used to produce the outcomes. In order to align the processes with the policies, an agency may have to completely reengineer its operating procedures. The old procedures for quality assurance (QA), for example, will have to be completely overhauled if prevention-based strategies are to be utilized. Subjective audits or other monitoring tools will have to be replaced with objective tools in monitoring the process of patient care and administration outcomes. A quantifiable method of determining the outcome of patient care will have to be used in order to determine the spread of variation within the process. The variables control charts are excellent tools for this purpose.

The last policy issue concerns measurement system data. In the past, the measurement system itself contributed to the problems inherent in improving quality. These systems could not distinguish between issues of accuracy and precision and were not capable of objectivity when using human sensors.

Accuracy and precision in the measurement system will determine the effectiveness and efficiency of the entire data system. The degree to which the measurement system provides valid information about the process under study will determine the effectiveness of the unit of measure. The determination and placement of the sensor will determine the accuracy and purpose of the measure. The degree to which the sensor is objective, reliable, and capable of replication will determine the precision of the system. Each of these issues are of extreme importance when developing the measurement system.

For example, look at Figure 3–2. The center target is neither accurate nor precise. The #2 target is an illustration of precision. In this case, the gun's site was slightly off, creating a precise shooting range, but it is not accurate. However, with a small adjustment, the shooter can get the effect shown in target #3, i.e., both precise and accurate.

The measurement system should focus on two types of data:

1. Process deficiencies focus internally and come from attributes data (decisions regarding good/bad, right/wrong). Generally, these data are found in error rates, failure rates, and other risk-prone incidents. Units of measure for process deficiencies are:

$$\text{Quality} = \frac{\text{frequency of deficiencies}}{\text{opportunities for deficiencies}}$$

2. Process features focus externally and come from units of measure that describe process output. These can be cycle-time, cost of quality, outcomes of care, ratio of bad debt to sales, etc. Units of measure for process features are real time measures showing output comparison to standard of performance. These are generally shown over time for improvement purposes.

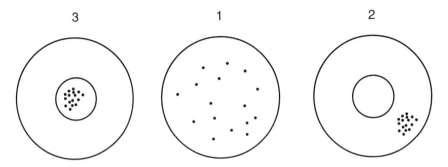

Figure 3–2 Transforming Units of Measure into Useful Information

The sensor, previously mentioned, can be a problem source for the measurement system. A sensor is defined as a method or tool designed to evaluate. Its accuracy depends on the degree to which the sensor is reflective of the purpose of the measure. A common problem with sensors is their placement within the process being measured. For example, an agency used the medical record as a sensor to evaluate a new nurse at 90 days posthire. This brings several issues to light:

- The medical record as a unit of measure is not precise. What part of the record will be reviewed, by what criteria, and over what period of time? All units of measure require precise definition. (We are back to the blue shirt story again!) If the word *error* is used in our definition, how do we define error?
- The placement of the evaluation tool (the medical record) 90 days posthire confuses what is being measured. Are we measuring the nurse's ability to document or are we measuring the nurse's retention of orientation information? Accuracy cannot be assured in this scenario.
- A supervisory nurse must review the medical record to make a judgment regarding its conformance to standards. There is no specificity regarding these standards. Therefore, this review will be subjective.

Juran maintains that "the precision of a sensor is a measure of the ability of the sensor to reproduce its results on a repeat test."[1] However, the *accuracy* of a sensor is the degree to which the sensor tells the truth. In the above example, it is unlikely that the sensor could be used by another nurse with exactly the same result.

It should also be noted that Juran looks at human sensors as "notoriously less precise than technological sensors."[2] There are, however, ways to remedy some of the problems in using human sensors. For example, misinterpretations can be remedied with precise and clear definitions of what to do, how to do it, by what means, under what criteria, using which documents, etc. Operational definition has been discussed earlier in this text and its principles apply here. Nothing must be left to chance when it comes to instruction.

No measurement system would be complete without representation of the two most important aspects for quality: (1) cost of quality and (2) customer-focused measures. As mentioned previously, the measurement system has externally focused process features as part of the real time measures. These process features should be the key quality characteristics discussed under CQI concept #7 (see Chapter 2). Additionally, the cost of quality measures should become the overall indicator of success for the TQM initiatives. As quality improves, costs go down. The overall cost of quality will begin to diminish as the quality efforts of agencies begin to pay off.

This is not to say, however, that quality is free, as Crosby would have us believe. CQI and TQM have associated up-front costs that will drive up the cost of quality for the first year or so. Expenditures on prevention and training are made simultaneously with maintaining the "old" way of doing business (with traditional inspection, for example). Costs will not begin to decrease until the training and prevention methods have begun to pay off. Crosby's "quality is free" referred to the long-term payback from quality improvement initiatives.[3] This payback is real and was proven in the General Accounting Office (GAO) study discussed in Chapter 2. The payback, however, will take time.

Education

It has been said that quality begins and ends with education. Two of Deming's 14 management points address the issue of education: (1) point 6: institute training on the job, and (2) point 13: institute a vigorous program of education.[4] It would seem at first glance that these two points are redundant. However, each addresses a different aspect of learning.

Point 6 refers to a systemic method whereby each employee can be trained in a consistent, effective, and productive manner. Most home care agencies have some type of on-the-job training program for new staff. This training generally includes a tenured aide accompanying a new home health aide (HHA) for a few days to "learn the ropes." The same is true for nurses. Office staff may or may not have someone accompany them while they learn the job, depending on turnover. This system has not proven effective, since on-the-job training lacks consistency. Different people are used as mentors or preceptors without benefit of knowledge in adult education. Also, these programs rarely have curriculum guides for core competencies and almost never have a system of credentialing post-training. On the other hand, these programs always seem to impart to new employees bad habits and shortcuts that may or may not be correct.

The on-the-job training addressed in point 6 establishes a program of certification for mentors or preceptors who have proven proficiency in the core competencies needed for the job. These mentors are prepared to deliver objective, consistent teaching in an effective manner. This type of training is always integrated with classroom training for initial delivery of course material. New employees can follow an established and consistent training course with proficiency testing at key points. On-the-job training becomes a systemic method for imparting knowledge about the job and the proficiencies required to do it.

Point 13 addresses education from a theoretical perspective. Learning has not taken place until theory is understood. The following story illustrates the point:

> A seagull swooped down and grabbed a clam off the sand. He flew high over the coast and dropped the clam on the sharp rocks below. The clam cracked open and the sea gull had lunch. A crow was watching the seagull all the while. Thinking this was an easy way to get a good lunch, he, too, swooped down and grabbed a clam from the sand. He flew high over the beach and dropped the clam on the sand. The clam dug his way into the sand and the crow went hungry.

This story teaches a valuable lesson. The crow mimicked the seagull but did not understand the theory behind dropping the clam on the rocks. Simply watching someone do something does not teach what is necessary. Employees must understand why they should do things in a certain way.

Deming's point 13 further implies that any self-improvement program, job related or not, will improve employee performance on the job.

An agency serious about TQM must initiate a rigorous training program in job-specific skills as well as in quality theory. It is interesting to note that training is one of the most important expenditures in world-class companies. In fact, these companies consider training an investment. Even in times of economic downturn, these companies do not cut back on training, as it is seen as the company's future. Also of note, these same companies almost always involve their highest-ranking officials in the actual delivery of training.

Example

This method of alignment is perhaps the most important. The example set by the leadership of the agency can make or break the quality initiatives. Senior leadership must convey to the staff the importance of quality not by what it says, but by what it does.

If branch managers are bonused on profitability, then profitability is what's important. If leadership talks of growth at management meetings, then growth is what's important. If leadership says quality is a given, then quality will not be achieved.

TQM as previously discussed, is about integrity. It is about alignment with the agency's mission, procedures, and practices. If the agency is serious about total quality, then it must be serious about doing the right thing for its customers and employees. If employees understand what to do, they will do it. For this reason, there can be no disconnects within the agency. There can be no contradictions, no mixed messages. Every action and communication must put forth the message that consistent conformance to customer expectations is required.

Figure 3–3 is an illustration of alignment and cascading effect. This cascading effect is also an approach to process reengineering, which is usually done synergistically with TQM.

The issue of alignment brings to mind the tragic events surrounding the Challenger disaster. The National Aeronautics and Space Administration (NASA) had a well-advertised mission that paraphrased, said, "safety first." The o-rings failed to meet design specifications, yet NASA continued to fly. Tremendous pressure was applied to NASA to fly missions on time every time. The disconnect occurred when the pressures became more important than the agency's mission of safety first.

Home health care providers are also exposed to great pressures. Pressures from the intermediary for utilization management and cost control; from insurance companies for discounts; from the patients for more services; from physicians for payments; from the public for indigent care; from the bankers for fiscal solvency; from employees for more money—pressures and more pressures.

TQM offers a method to prioritize these pressures for the long-term success of the agency, i.e., to provide ever-improving value to customers. Drucker said that long-term thinking allows you to mold your own future by understanding the consequences of today's decisions.[5] He goes on to say that decision makers should face up to reality and resist the temptation of what "everybody knows."

Today's decisions, using a TQM methodology, must be made in accordance with the mission and vision of the agency with all other operational aspects in full alignment.

BRIDGE TO THE FUTURE

The use of TQM in home care discussed in this book will accomplish the goal all of us share, improved outcomes of care. It will also become the foundation for growth and further opportunity as our industry enters the twenty-first century.

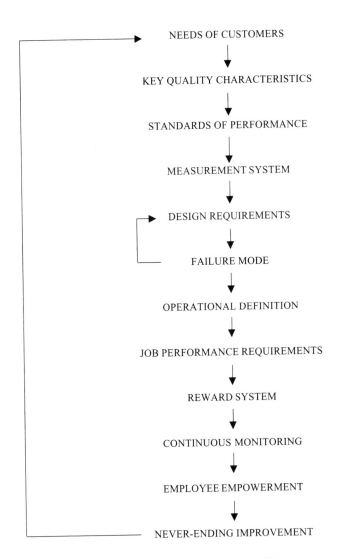

Figure 3–3 Illustration of Alignment and Cascading Effect

The decade of the 1990s will be a challenge for those with the vision to build bridges to the future. Those bridges will be built upon a foundation of quality and productivity. Our job has just begun.

NOTES

1. J.M. Juran, *Juran on Quality by Design* (The Free Press, New York: The Juran Institute, Inc., 1992), p. 126.

2. Ibid., p. 130.

3. P.B. Crosby, *Quality Is Free, the Art of Making Quality Certain* (New York: Penguin Group, 1980).

4. W.E. Deming, *Out of Crisis* (Cambridge, Mass.: Massachusetts Institute of Technology, 1982).

5. P.F. Drucker, *Managing in Turbulent Times* (New York: Harper & Row Publishers, 1980), p. 5.

Chapter 4

Customer Relationships

WHO IS THE CUSTOMER?

"Consistent conformance to customer expectations with minimal variation"—this definition says all that needs to be said regarding the connection between quality and customer relationships. Customers are the ultimate determining factor in quality and whether or not an agency will stay in business. Deming's first point is constancy of purpose, which means to constantly improve the quality of services. This, in turn, ensures remaining in business and continuing to provide jobs.

Who is the customer? Although the customer is many people, for purposes of this discussion the customer will be defined as anyone to whom work is given or who receives benefit from work performed, e.g., patients, clients, referral sources, physicians, government, management, and employees. In home care, customers can be segmented into three basic categories:

1. Primary customers (end users or those who order end use):
   - patients
   - families
   - physicians
   - referral sources
2. Secondary customers (those who pay for or regulate services):
   - payer sources
   - regulators
   - standards groups
   - managed care groups
3. Auxiliary customers (those who have a vested interest in the services):
   - employees
   - supervisors

- suppliers
- contractors
- stockholders

Each of these customer segments has different needs and expectations, while each subgroup may also have differences regarding its needs. A broad generalization of the breakdown between these segments follows:

1. Primary customers are the ultimate downstream customer, referred to as the end user. Primary customers are also those who order end use.
2. Secondary customers are those who pay for end use or those who regulate end use.
3. Auxiliary customers are internal customers who have a vested interest in the success of the agency. These could be employees, suppliers, and contractors.

Exhibit 4–1 defines the customer segments.

Deming defined quality as meeting customers' needs at a price they are willing to pay. This definition has two components: customers' needs and the price they are willing to pay.

THE CUSTOMER'S NEEDS

There are three levels of needs that every customer has when he or she seeks home care or is otherwise involved in ordering, paying for, regulating, or providing the service. These needs classifications are:

Exhibit 4–1 Customer Segments

PRIMARY CUSTOMERS	SECONDARY CUSTOMERS	AUXILIARY CUSTOMERS
Patients	Payer Sources	Employees
Families	Regulators	Supervisors
Physicians	Standards Groups	Suppliers
Referrals	Managed Care Providers	Contractors
		Stockholders

1. Specifications—"I need"
2. Expectations—"I want"
3. Unexpected added value—"I wish"

Each of these classifications can be explored in detail (see Figure 4–1).

Specifications

The specifications are the primary reason a customer will pick up the phone to call for home care. This need category should be considered absolute. In other words, the agency must meet this criterion or risk losing the patient. Specifications offer little room for maneuvering, although there is generally some room for negotiating. In order for the specification to be met to the satisfaction of all parties, an operational definition of the specification must be agreed to in advance of the service. Without this level of specificity, the agency is in the dark regarding the real specification.

For example, a physician may call and order home care for a patient for daily dressing changes for seven days. The physician will see the patient at the end of the first week and decide on the continued treatment plan at that time. Insurance verification confirms coverage. The agency believes all is well and proceeds to render care. On the third day of treatment, the regular registered nurse (RN) who has been seeing the patient calls in sick and the only person available is a licensed practical nurse (LPN), who changes the dressing. The physician sees the patient at the end of the first week and is upset that the wound has not improved as desired. The physician calls the agency to ask the enterostomal therapist (ET) what technique was used. The physician is furious to find that an ET did not see the patient at all and, as a result, discharges the patient from care. If this is not bad enough, the agency bills the insurance company and is denied the visit made by the LPN. This coverage will pay only for services of an RN.

Figure 4–1 Customer's Needs Classifications

This difficult situation could have been avoided if the agency had been proficient in defining the operational definition of the specification. In this type of case, the intake nurse should have asked the physician if he wanted an ET. Likewise, the parameters should have been set with the insurance company regarding whether coverage was for RNs only or for any level of skilled nursing.

As this example illustrates, specifications are different for every customer. In order to meet the specifications of all customers involved, detailed questions must be asked. Probing the caller for operational definition requires a skill that comes with practice.

It should also be mentioned that while many nurses are adept at gleaning operational definition from physicians as a result of their training in the specifics of recording physician's orders, they almost always fail to exercise the same caution with the patient. The probable cause, again, is training. Nurses have not been trained by the profession to respond to a patient as the "controller" of the service. Continuous quality improvement puts the patient in a controlling position equal to that of the physician.

Specifications are articulated requirements of each customer group which must be consistently met. Failure to perform satisfactorily on a specified requirement results in a reliability crisis.

Professors Zeithami, Parasuraman, and Berry of Texas A&M University developed a model for dimensions of customer service rated by relative importance. In their book, *Delivering Quality Service*, the professors explain that reliability is the most important service attribute, followed in order of importance by responsiveness, assurance of quality, empathy, and intangibles.

A client who was using a home care agency to provide after-school care for her Down syndrome child experienced a reliability crisis when the caregiver failed to show up one afternoon. The mother was not notified and the special school the child attended dropped him off as usual at his home. The child, who had the cognitive ability of a four-year-old was left alone for approximately three hours. You can imagine the trauma the mother experienced when she returned home from work to find her child had been left alone.

This scenario exemplifies a reliability crisis. Customers will perceive failures in this area as major problems. For this reason, reliability issues will always be a key quality characteristic. Agency administrators will do well to make issues of reliability a top priority.

Expectations

The expectations of customers can be broken down into two categories:

- expectations that are stated
- expectations that are implied

Stated expectations are those that customers say that want, but they will rarely leave the agency if these expectations are not met consistently. On the other hand, if the agency never meets these expectations, patients will tend to go elsewhere. For example, the patient's stated expectation is for the home health aide (HHA) to come at 8:00 A.M. on Monday, Wednesday, and Friday. If the aide is occasionally late or needs to reschedule because of a holiday, the patient will generally continue to accept the service. If, on the other hand, the aide ignores the patient's expectations and always comes at different times and on different days, the patient may go to another agency.

Expectations that are implied are very similar to Herzberg's two-factor theory discussed in Chapter 6. Herzberg's theory of satisfaction was based on motivators and demotivators. The demotivators did not contribute to satisfaction, but their absence led to dissatisfaction. The same is true for implied expectations. In other words, if the agency fails to meet an implied expectation, dissatisfaction will result. On the other hand, even if the agency consistently meets the implied expectations, satisfaction is not increased.

For example, the client has an implied expectation that the nurse will come to the home with a clean uniform. If the nurse complies (and has on a clean uniform) the issue stays subliminal. If, however, the nurse shows up wearing a dirty uniform, the client will be dissatisfied.

To further complicate this category of customer expectations, the implied expectations will almost never be in conscious thought and therefore will not be expressed as an expectation. It also should be pointed out that each of these categories of expectations will require operational definition before the agency attempts to meet them.

Expectations, stated or implied, are requirements that, like specifications, must be consistently met in order to satisfy customers. Failure to meet an expectation results in "points" being taken away from the relationship experience.

Unexpected Added Value

This category of customer needs is quite possibly the most important, for meeting these needs will have the effect of setting industry standards. This group of needs can best be described as the "desire" or "wish" characteristics of service. Like the subliminal implied expectations, this group of needs also is unarticulated by the customer segments.

This group of needs is hard to describe because few people in today's busy world take the time to dream "what if" about the services they use.

Federal Express is an excellent example of a company that was able to set operational definition to the added value features of its service. No one in its industry was able to guarantee 10:30 A.M. delivery until Federal Express committed to doing so. Its business customers did not expect this level of service and were delighted. Business boomed and the Federal Express market share grew. As the customers got 10:30 A.M. delivery consistently, this added value changed to a stated expectation. This is the point at which Federal Express set the industry standard. Today, the expectation has moved to a specification, and the entire industry must meet this need in order to stay competitive.

The added value features of customer service is the fluid need category. In other words, as this need is consistently met, it will move into the expectation category (industry standard), and over time will come to rest in the specification category. The key to the fluid movement of the added value category is consistency. If the added value feature is not consistently applied to the service as a whole, it will continue to be wonderful when it happens, but the customers will not come to depend on it. Without this dependence, customers will not guarantee their loyalty. Building customer loyalty is dependent upon added value services that can be translated into key quality characteristics. For purposes of this discussion, added value services are those that were not specified or expected. Unexpected added value will delight customers and help build the loyalty necessary for long-term relationships.

Figure 4–1 illustrates the relationship of the needs classifications to the customer's willingness to pay.

THE PRICE THE CUSTOMER WILL PAY

Customers pay for a service based on their perception of its value to them. If the service offered by the agency is perceived as valuable to customers, and the service consistently meets all of their needs, a customer will pay a premium price and have the perception of value. On the other hand, if the service does not consistently meet the customers' needs, they will not be willing to pay a higher price nor will they perceive value.

Consistency in the service delivery component of the agency's business is the key to customer service and relationship building. If the service is excellent one day and average the next time, customers will become disillusioned and not know what to expect. Customers tend to remember the last encounter, so make sure it is a positive one.

A last note on pricing concerns agencies who have a predominance of Medicare patients. These agencies have paid little or no attention to the issue of price. With the competition increasing for the private-pay client and with prospective payment looming, agency administrators will do well to pay closer attention to this issue in the future.

There is a direct relationship between price and the perceived value of the service. The willingness to pay is based on the perceived value the service has to the customer. Customer research has indicated that generally, customers are not overwhelmingly satisfied with the price they pay for services. However, in companies that have good reputations for service, the satisfaction rating on value for price is significantly higher.

The relationship with customers does not suffer if customers perceive that the value they received was worth the price they paid. Without this perception, the relationship will suffer. This can create hostility in customers who feel "ripped off."

In addition to the different customer segments and the different needs classifications, there are distinct differences between internal and external customers. The external customers are the primary and secondary groups, while the internal customers are classified as the auxiliary group.

Employee Expectations

What are the employee's expectations? Is the agency meeting those expectations? If the answer to either of these questions is no, the employees may not be as satisfied with their employment as desired. Employees who are not satisfied do not excel nor do they generally stay. Turnover is expensive in lost productivity, training, and recruitment costs. Satisfied employees, on the other hand, tend to stay longer and to display better productivity and compliance with standards. Research has proven that there is a direct correlation between employee satisfaction and customer satisfaction. Many companies have come to believe that the way they treat their employees will be the way the employees treat their customers. It is for these reasons that agencies should do all they can to ensure the satisfaction of their employees.

Obviously, the agency's intent should be to retain valued employees. An employee questionnaire can help to determine the expectations of the staff by establishing some baseline data. It is important to have baseline data in order to ascertain whether there are any issues that are consistent with all or a majority of employees. For example, a majority of employees may respond that they would like to see dental insurance added to the company's benefits package. In this case, the agency should make every effort to comply. On the other hand, maybe only one or two older employees asked for a pension plan. This benefit, therefore, is not important to the majority of employees.

The employee questionnaire is a helpful tool in determining perceptions of management attitudes, which is an important aspect of employee morale and satisfaction. It should be emphasized that this questionnaire is not for the purpose of discipline; rather, it is intended to develop better understanding and relationships between staff and management. The questionnaire will also identify whether employees understand and accept the agency's goals and objectives. Exhibit 4–2 provides an example of an employee questionnaire.

Remember, the purpose of the questionnaire is to improve the relationship of staff to the management of the agency and to ultimately improve the satisfaction of employees by responding to their stated needs (expectations). In order for the purpose to be accomplished, however, management must LISTEN and RE-SPOND.[1] Agency management must understand that listening to employees and

---

Exhibit 4–2 Employee Questionnaire

Discipline _____

Branch   _____

1. What is the thing you like *best* about the agency?

2. What is the thing you like *least* about the agency?

3. Do you believe you are held totally accountable for your job responsibilities?

4. Do you believe it is okay to make mistakes?

5. How does the agency respond to mistakes?

6. Do you and your colleagues work well as a team when necessary?

7. What would you like to see the agency do to improve employee morale?

8. How do you think the agency can improve on quality?

9. Do you believe internal problems are resolved in an open manner?

10. What would you like to get out of your association with the agency?

11. The corporate mission statement is:

Exhibit 4–2 continued

"Enhancing the quality of life through the delivery of compassionate health care at home by skilled professionals continuously striving for excellence"

What do you think of that statement?

_____

12. Please state the agency's goals.

_____

13. How are you committed to the agency's success?

_____

14. Are you genuinely willing to try new things?

_____

_____

15. Do you believe there is a high degree of mutual respect or trust between people employed here?

_____

_____

16. Do you believe that finding the truth is more important than being right in this agency?

_____

17. Do you believe the pay and benefits are adequate?

_____

18. What pay and benefits would you like deleted or added?

_____

19. Do you believe the incentive programs are sufficient to motivate you?

_____

20. Tell us about your most satisfying experience at the agency.

_____

_____

21. Tell us about your least satisfying experience at the agency.

_____

_____

understanding what they are really saying is only half the expectation. The other half is the response. Each employee should be given the results of the questionnaire and told how management intends to respond to concerns or issues raised.

As stated previously, this type of questionnaire is an open-ended survey format designed to elicit responses about the relationship between employees and management. This type of survey instrument, however, will not provide the information needed to develop key quality characteristics for employees or to design process improvement. This type of survey instrument requires an events-based model, which will be discussed in detail later in this chapter.

Another excellent opportunity to listen and respond to employees is the old-fashioned, but highly useful, suggestion program. Employees know better ways of accomplishing tasks and should be encouraged to share their ideas. An award should be given to any employee who contributes a suggestion that improves the agency's operations. These innovative employees should be recognized and rewarded for their contributions. All employees should be familiar with contributed suggestions and management responses to them. A sample of suggestions and responses is provided as an example:

Suggestion: Please consider the amount of mileage driven as com-
              pared to productivity (it's not fair to ask someone to drive
              80–110 miles and see the same number of patients as
              someone who drives 30–50 miles).
Response: Excessive mileage is taken into consideration on a monthly
              average and figured into the productivity ratios. Someone
              who drives over the 70-mile standard has his or her
              number of patients reduced.
Suggestion: Try an RN flowsheet to keep a record of procedures and
              dates to be performed (would be helpful to PRN nurses).
Response: There is currently a procedure for PRN nurses to update
              them about the patients they are asked to see; however,
              the case managers are not following this procedure.
              Discuss with the branch manager and follow up with
              administrator if necessary.
Suggestion: Adopt as abbreviations: Inst = instructed; demo = dem-
              onstration; I/S = instruct/supervise.
Response: Accepted. $10 earned.

The Japanese have a system called Kaizen that, loosely translated, means small incremental improvements. This system has found its way into the more traditional employee suggestion programs in the United States. American business leaders have followed the Toyota Corporation's approach of strongly encouraging employees to suggest small improvements to their work. The result has been a greater involvement in the improvement initiatives. Employee involvement is an indicator of morale and well-being and should be tracked for the quality improvement program.

Other recognition and awards or rewards should be standard operating procedure within the agency. Employees want most to be recognized and rewarded for outstanding achievement. This process sets up the role models and "superstars" for all other employees to emulate. Awards should be designed carefully, however, and the tools of continuous quality improvement should be used to determine the superstars.

It has been recognized that employees stay with companies for reasons other than money. High on the list for staying are job satisfaction and recognition.

Recognition Program

A proposed program for recognition of exemplary performance and conduct would include the prominent display in each office of a large poster board bearing the names of employees and significant contractors. The display board should be broken down as shown in Exhibit 4–3.

The categories for tracking employee recognition under this program are suggestions for improvement, patient/client compliments, and outstanding achievement.

Suggestions for Improvement. It is important that each employee and contractor understand that management values their ideas and suggestions. A suggestion

---

Exhibit 4–3 Employee Recognition Tracking

Name	Suggestions for Improvement	Patient/Client Compliments	Outstanding Achievement (for growth or quality)

box should be placed in every office for easy access to employees and caregivers. Suggestions by employees should be actively encouraged, since encouragement shows that management is interested in their ideas. These suggestions should always be for the purpose of improvement, whether it be in patient care, operations, or financial savings.

When an employee makes a suggestion for improvement, place a red star on the board for all to see. Also, recognize this employee at staff meetings or other gatherings to reinforce positive behavior.

Patient/Client Compliments. The heart of the home care business is a good relationship with patients, clients, and other customers. Staff should know that a compliment from an outside source is the best form of public relations. Every employee is encouraged to do the kind of work that someone would want to compliment. When a compliment is received, place a red star next to the person's name and again, recognize the employee at a meeting.

Outstanding Achievements. The key to the success of the home care business is growth coupled with quality. The business cannot succeed without both. Management wants to recognize employees for outstanding achievement in the areas of either growth, or quality, or both! When an employee has performed in an exemplary fashion, place a gold star on the superstar chart. Make sure the stars are always based on quantifiable results. This will keep the program from turning into a popularity contest. Additionally, these employees should have a commendation written by the manager and placed in their permanent record, with a copy to the regional manager if applicable.

At the end of each period (month, quarter, or year), the employee with the most stars in each category is given a certificate or plaque in honor of being one of the agency's superstars.

Experience has shown that the program costs little or nothing, yet brings tremendous satisfaction to employees.

Employee Exit Interview Questionnaire

Another valuable, but often overlooked, tool for increased employee satisfaction is the employee exit interview questionnaire. This questionnaire was designed as a personal interview of an employee who is leaving the agency but can also double as the employee questionnaire. It is critical to the success of employee relations to ascertain the reasons why a staff member chooses to leave the agency. Valuable trends can be established that can help the agency identify and correct problems before others choose to leave. An example of this type of questionnaire appears in Exhibit 4–4.

All the questionnaires in the world will do no good toward improving employee relations if the results are not shared and, most importantly, acted

Exhibit 4–4 Employee Exit Interview Questionnaire—Staff Member Evaluation of Employment (Strictly Confidential)

We are dedicated to providing satisfying employment for all personnel. Please complete this form so we can better measure how well we have provided satisfying employment for you and how we can improve. Thank you.

Name _____ Discipline _____ Branch _____

	Agree	Do Not Agree	Comments
1. My work was interesting to me.			
2. I was encouraged to take initiatives in my work.			
3. I was encouraged to make suggestions about my work.			
4. My work gave me a chance to use my knowledge and skills.			
5. I had sufficient time to keep up with my work.			
6. I approved of my work assignments.			
7. I was given sufficient instruction regarding my work assignments.			
8. I was given sufficient information about situations that might affect my work.			
9. The orientation program I participated in was sufficient.			
10. The education programs I participated in were sufficient.			
11. The home health care agency atmosphere seemed to be one of cooperation.			
12. Adequate equipment was available for performing my work tasks.			

continues

Exhibit 4–4 continued

	Agree	Do Not Agree	Comments
13. Adequate career advancement opportunities were available to me.			
14. Sufficient personnel benefits were available to me.			
15. My salary compared favorably with salaries elsewhere for comparable work.			
16. The home health care agency management staff were fair with me concerning agency policies and procedures.			
17. The home health care agency management staff sufficiently dealt with staff members' concerns and problems.			
18. I felt comfortable in asking questions of the home health care agency management staff.			
19. I felt comfortable voicing concerns and problems to the home health care agency management staff.			
20. I felt my immediate supervisor supported me.			
21. I plan to continue working in home health care.			
22. I felt the office support staff were helpful to me.			
23. My peers were helpful to me in my job.			

24. Additional comments:

_____

_____

_____

Exhibit 4-4 continued

25. Your position title: _____

26. Your length of employment: _____

27. Your reason(s) for leaving: _____
_____
_____

28. What steps could have been taken that would have prevented your leaving?
_____

29. Type of position you may seek/have obtained (if applicable): _____
_____

30. How does it compare to the one you are leaving? _____

31. Would you recommend employment with the home health care agency to a friend as a good place to work?

    _____ Yes _____ No

    Please explain: _____
    _____
    _____
    _____

32. When you started your job, were you informed of your duties, hours of work, pay rate, immediate supervisor, etc.? _____
    _____
    _____
    _____
    _____

upon. This includes changing the processes necessary to help staff perform better.

Management Expectations

The first rule of management is to understand that the manager works for the employee. It is the job of managers to support and reinforce employee expectations of the agency, the profession, and staff working relationships. Managers of home health care agencies should know that an overwhelming majority of jobs today are in the service industry. The biggest problem managers face is that some employees in the service field do not look upon their jobs as important. It is the manager's responsibility to make each employee understand the importance of the employee's individual role, both in the overall corporate structure and for quality improvement.

Recognition is one way a manager can impart to employees the importance of each job and to recognize that level of importance in various and meaningful ways.

Each person should know the standards by which he or she is judged. This component has been discussed in almost every chapter of this book. Managers should share the audit tools with employees, train on them, and use them for developmental purposes. A manager is responsible to the employees to ensure they know the agency's standards. The employees will be in a position to self-measure their progress toward meeting those standards. The Deming model addresses this issue as quality continuation—the process by which self-measurement is possible. Employees can measure their own performance by utilizing the same audit tools that management will use. Employees should be trained in the tools of continuous quality improvement and assisted in their use as the method by which self-measurement is quantified.

Referral Source Expectations

Referral source expectations are external expectations. The same questions asked under employee expectations should be asked of referral sources. The same answers also apply. Determining referral source expectations may encompass some surprises.

For example, a survey asked 27 hospital discharge planners to rank in order of importance the following issues:

- quality
- price
- service delivery

Instead of ranking quality as the most important, as was presumed, they ranked service delivery as the most important by 54 percent. Quality ranked second at 40 percent, and price was third with only 6 percent.

While this was an interesting insight into what this group of referral sources thought was the most important aspect of home care, their response to another question should also be considered. When asked whether home care accreditation was important to them, 90 percent of the respondents said yes, naming quality as their reason. This response was expected. Taken together, the responses to both issues make it clear that the agency's marketing efforts should be geared to service delivery with a strong emphasis on quality. This marketing strategy, which combines the most important issues identified by this group of respondents, was remarkably successful. In October of 1988, when the survey was first conducted, the agency was doing 5,600 visits per month. By October of 1989, the agency did 10,640 visits a month—a startling 52 percent increase in visits in just one year!

Determining Expectations

When an agency is able to meet the customer's expectations, growth is the natural outcome. Determining what those expectations are is the critical issue. An agency may want to consider different types of questionnaires or surveys: an evaluation of the agency's services, a customer questionnaire, and an events-based survey.

Evaluation of the Agency's Services. This questionnaire is designed to elicit responses from discharge planners or social workers in hospitals regarding satisfaction with services rendered by the agency. It is suggested this survey be done at least annually by person-to-person contact. This exercise also indicates the agency's willingness to listen and take action on the concerns of key referral sources.

The following questions are open-ended in order to get the social worker or discharge planer to talk about the response. This also gives the interviewer the opportunity to respond in a positive manner. For this reason, it is recommended that the highest ranking official at the agency conduct this survey. Some examples of questions for a discharge planner questionnaire are:

1. How would you rate the overall service delivery of the agency?
2. Based on your feedback from patients and physicians, how would you rate the agency?
3. Based on your interactions with our staff, how would you rate the professionalism and performance of our staff?
4. When telephoning our agency, have you been satisfied with the staff's response?
5. Were you satisfied with the way you were kept informed of the patient's condition?
6. Would you recommend this agency to other patients in your facility?
7. Do you have any comments or suggestions on ways we can provide better service?
8. Have you ever experienced a problem with this agency? If so, explain.

Customer Questionnaire. This tool was developed as a means of determining the expectations of key referral sources of home care in general, and specifically where the agency is in relation to those expectations. This survey should be conducted by someone not associated with the agency nor identified as conducting the survey on the agency's behalf. The questionnaire serves the purpose of determining the agency's market position within the community. Additionally, it can help the agency identify the issues on which to focus during marketing and advertising efforts. An example of this survey tool is provided in Exhibit 4–5.

This questionnaire is open-ended in order to allow the referral source to respond in any manner without the predetermined prejudices of categorization. For example, in conducting this survey, the agency found that for social workers, the definition of quality was absence of complaints. While the agency believed that quality would be the most important attribute, the survey proved that service delivery was the most important. This type of questionnaire can be extremely valuable in formulating a long-range plan for the growth and development of the agency.

Physician Evaluation Questionnaire. Another type of questionnaire under referral source is the evaluation tool for physicians. This questionnaire identifies physicians' feelings about the agency's services. This questionnaire should be given to all referring physicians at least annually or upon discharge of individual physicians' clients. The results of this questionnaire should be included in the agency's annual evaluation. Some sample questions appear in Exhibit 4–6.

Client Expectations

There has been a great deal written lately regarding patient or customer satisfaction. Prior to the late 1980s, patient or client satisfaction was not an issue to which much thought was given by health care professionals. With today's emphasis on quality improvement, the recipient of health care plays a paramount role in determining who will be the provider of health care. That decision rests largely with the public's perception of quality. The general public is not in a position to know which provider is the most technically competent or which home care agency has the best results or outcome criteria.

The public, however, is in a position to know and respond to providers who treat people with sensitivity, courtesy, respect, and friendliness. These are the ingredients for customer satisfaction in any business. Quality is, for the most part, presumed when the customer has been treated with kindness, compassion, and courtesy and when his or her needs have been met.

A good example of this hypothesis is the lawyer who will say that the filing of a malpractice suit depends largely on the way the patient was treated.

Exhibit 4–5 Customer Questionnaire

Customer _____   Date _____

Interviewee _____   Position _____

Interviewer _____

1. How do you define quality?
2. Specify your needs in home care:
3. Please rank in order of importance the following:

   quality/price/service delivery
4. How would you improve the home care industry?
5. Of all the home care providers, please name the one that, in your opinion, has the best reputation in the following areas:

   Quality _____

   Service delivery _____

   Best trained nurses _____

   Most helpful when you call _____

   Goes above and beyond _____

   Can handle difficult patients _____

   Private duty _____
6. What do you like best about the following agencies (list local agencies):

   _____

   _____

   _____

   _____
7. What do you like least about these agencies (list local agencies):

   _____

   _____

   _____

   _____
8. Is there a specific service you would like to see started by home care providers?
9. Is accreditation by the Joint Commission on Accreditation of Healthcare Organizations important to you?

   If so, why?
10. How are you meeting the home care needs of indigent patients?
11. How are your potential recipients of home care educated about the industry?
12. What would you tell American Association of Retired Persons members to look for when choosing a home care agency?

Exhibit 4–6 Physician Evaluation Questionnaire

Dear Dr. _____

In an effort to continually improve our agency, we would appreciate your answering a few questions relative to the service we have given your patients. Your answers will be used as part of our agency's annual evaluation.

EVALUATION QUESTIONNAIRE

1. How would you rate the professionalism of our nursing staff?
   Excellent _____   Good _____
   Fair _____   Poor _____
2. How would you rate the overall performance of our staff?
   Excellent _____   Good _____
   Fair _____   Poor _____
3. Were you satisfied with the way in which you have been kept apprised of your patient's condition?
   Excellent _____   Good _____
   Fair _____   Poor _____
4. Would you recommend the agency to others?
   Excellent _____   Good _____
   Fair _____   Poor _____
5. Do you have any comments or suggestions on ways in which we can provide a better service?

Thank You.

Branch Manager _____   Physician's Signature _____

A different example is the patient who went for her first mammogram. She went to a hospital outpatient clinic for the test, and upon entering was ushered into a large reception room staffed by several clerks in front of computer terminal screens. At each desk a client gave confidential information, including medical information, to a clerk, who typed it into the computer. She was able to overhear everything said by two other clients nearest to her. She was appalled by the lack of privacy and felt completely ill at ease. Needless to say, when the annual mammogram rolled around again, the patient found a different provider.

In July, 1989, Ericksen wrote that the

> . . . relationship between quality of nursing care and patient satisfaction
> . . . indicates an inverse relationship for the most part. This suggests that
> nurses should be cautious in equating patient satisfaction with quality
> of nurse care.[2]

Ericksen's thesis was that patients were not happy going through the difficulties of treatment, e.g., blood draws, catheter insertions, changes in diet, etc., that are necessitated by good nursing practice. However, her study did show a direct relationship between patient satisfaction and the social courtesy they received. This study and others suggest that though patients are subjected to uncomfortable procedures, if the nurse is informative, considerate, kind, and compassionate, the patient will still feel a sense of satisfaction.

A telephone call-back system was successfully instituted in Ohio. Nurses called back each patient who was treated. The objectives of this program were to:

1. enhance the patient's perception about quality of care
2. provide an opportunity for patients to have questions answered or make additional referrals as necessary
3. enable the nurse to have an enlightened perspective on the common problems postdischarge
4. provide a final evaluation of the quality of care received by the discharged patient.

This one personal phone call by the nurse conveyed concern and caring and patients loved it!

Post Discharge Follow-Up Program

For home care, the telephone call-back system can be modified. The postdischarge follow-up program can determine the client's satisfaction and be a source of future referrals. All clients discharged from the agency could be called within 30 days of discharge to determine how they are doing currently and whether any further assistance is required. Findings are that patients and clients appreciate the thoughtfulness of agency personnel and this call enhances the customer's perception of the agency's quality. Clients are again called at intervals of 60 to 90 days to determine whether any new problems have been identified.

Experience has determined that the program can bring 10 to 15 percent of formally discharged patients and clients back as readmissions. This program should be administered by a staff member with at least the qualifications of an LPN who can call physicians for orders to evaluate when a problem is identified. Because of the readmission rate, the program can pay for itself. The program is simple to follow. Each client or patient has a post discharge form filled out at the time of discharge. This form is forwarded to the discharge nurse who suspends the form for 30 days, at which time follow-up begins. A sample form (Exhibit 4–7) and a summary (recap) form (Exhibit 4–8) for the overall program are provided.

Exhibit 4–7 Post Discharge and Nonadmit Follow-Up

Branch _____

Patient's Name _____   Phone _____

Address _____

Primary payment source _____

Date of discharge or nonadmit _____

Reason for discharge or nonadmit _____
_____

Diagnosis _____

Physician name at discharge or nonadmit _____ Phone _____

Date patient questionnaire sent _____ (Discharge)

Date nonadmission letter sent _____ (Nonadmit)

= =

Dates of Follow-Up

(First contact: 30 days Post discharge or Nonadmit)

Services Not Needed at This Time	Patient Expired	Requires Service*	Unable To Locate	No Answer	Do Not Call Again	Another HH Agency or SNF†

*Patient's condition/problems: _____

†HH = home health; SNF = skilled nursing facility.

Comments _____

Readmitting date _____

Suspense/60 days _____   Follow-up discharge nurse _____

Suspense/90 days _____

Exhibit 4-8 Post Discharge Program Recap

Branch _____

Fiscal Year _____

Follow-Up Discharge Nurse _____

	May	June	July	Aug	Sept	Oct	Nov	Dec	Jan	Feb	Mar	Apr	Year End Totals
(1) Total number of patients in discharge program ending previous months													
(2) Total number of discharges current month													
(3) Number of patients with final disposition:													
Expired													
ICF/SNF*													
Service not needed													
Unable to locate													
Do not call again													
Another home health agency													
Total													

continues

Exhibit 4-8 continued

	May	June	July	Aug	Sept	Oct	Nov	Dec	Jan	Feb	Mar	Apr	Year End Totals
(4) Number of patients readmitted													
(5) Total number of patients still receiving follow up													
Estimated amount of time spent this month on D/C* program													

Formula: #1
           + #2
           − #3
           − #4
           = Total that will become #5 (next month's #1)

*D/C = discharge; ICF = intermediate care facility; SNF = skilled nursing facility.

Events-Based Questionnaires

Throughout the discussion of questionnaires or surveys, many suggestions have been made to assist the agency in determining overall satisfaction. Samples have been provided for agencies to elicit customer responses to assist in improving customer relationships. However, there is another survey that can assist the agency in changing procedures in response to customer research. This research instrument uses an events-based model. This model should be applied by the more advanced agencies in the use of continuous quality improvement (CQI) tools and techniques. Briefly, the model works in the following manner:

1. All agency processes are flowcharted at Level 1.
2. Each process flowchart is color-coded based on the interaction between the task and a specific customer segment.
3. All like-colored tasks (representing interactions with a specific customer segment) are placed on a matrix set up with the vertical axis representing events such as scheduling, service delivery, etc. The horizontal axis represents each customer segment.
4. Indicate each task under each major event where an interaction takes place on the matrix for all customers combined. For example, scheduling is an event that has a task of arranging for a visit time. In this case, the scheduling coordinator as well as the patient and caregiver are involved. The matrix will have an X mark under each of these customer segments. This process allows the user to identify issues to address for each of the customer surveys.
5. Using the matrix, develop questions about specific interactions with each customer segment. For example, the last time I was contacted by the scheduler, I was pleased with her ability to arrange the visit at my convenience. Responses should be forced. In other words, write the survey in such a way as to force the respondent to answer in a certain category. In this example, responses could be: strongly agree; agree; mildly agree; neutral; mildly disagree; disagree; or strongly disagree.
6. Develop the questionnaire around major events such as scheduling; initial contact; admissions; receiving services; calling the office; billing; quality; etc. The opening question under each major category should be:

   > Overall, I am satisfied with the manner in which the agency handles scheduling.

   The "overall" questions become the dependent variables in each category.
7. After the overall question, ask specific questions regarding each of the major aspects of the event. In the case of scheduling, some issues to address include:

- convenience of the schedule
- advance notice
- changes in scheduling
- changes in the caregiver
- frequency and duration

Each of these questions become independent variables. These variables will cause the dependent variable (the overall question) to change for the better or worse depending on the response.

8. Use a computer program that will conduct multiple regression analysis. This type of analysis will assist the agency in identifying the key drivers of satisfaction or the key quality characteristics. These are the issues that will be the most important to customers.

The use of this type of detailed survey provides the foundation for process reengineering and other process improvement opportunities. These surveys are more complicated than the open-ended questions and should be undertaken by someone who has experience with these techniques.

Client Satisfaction Index

All these survey tools notwithstanding, the highest priority for any agency should be the satisfaction of current clients. Remember, quality is the customer's perception of how well the agency complied with his or her expectations. For this reason, the client satisfaction index (CSI) has been developed. This type of indexing will offer agency managers the objective data necessary to determine the areas of concern where improvement is necessary.

While the CSI can be used as a single tool it is most effective when coupled with other forms to assure the client of the agency's desire to conform to the customer's expectations. Such other forms may include, but not be limited to, the following:

1. "I care" card from the executive director or regional director that is given to every patient or client at the initial start of care (SOC). This card can be utilized by clients at any time they feel a problem is not being resolved at the local branch office level. A sample is provided in Exhibit 4–9.
2. "How are we doing" letter from the branch manager two weeks after care has started. The purpose of this letter is to establish contact between the local manager and client or patient for problem resolution with field or other staff. A sample is provided in Exhibit 4–10.

Both of these forms offer local management the opportunity to correct any problems while the client is being served by the agency.

Exhibit 4–9 "I Care" Card

I really do care! I care about the service you are receiving and I want it to be absolutely the *best*! If at any time during your treatment you feel things are not going as you think they should—*tell me*! Let me try to make things right for you.

If, on the other hand, you are well pleased with your care, I would like to know that, too. Please write to me on this card if there is anything at all I can do for you to make your care better. Thank you for your cooperation.

Executive Director

Comments: _____

_____

_____

_____

_____

Signed _____

Telephone Number

Exhibit 4–10 "How Are We Doing" Letter

Dear _____,

We are pleased you have chosen our agency to serve you during this period of illness or injury. It is our desire to meet your medical service needs to the best of our ability. Therefore, if there is anything we can do to improve our service to you, please so indicate on the bottom of this letter and return it to our office.

We are also interested in your comments on how we are doing so far in meeting your needs. Won't you please take a few minutes and respond in order that we may better serve you? You may return your response in the self-addressed, stamped envelope enclosed.

Sincerely,

_____

Branch Manager

Phone: _____

COMMENTS:
How are we doing so far?

_____

_____

How can we better serve you?

_____

_____

The CSI is the final step in the process to assure client satisfaction. Every client should be sent a client evaluation questionnaire at the time of discharge. The purpose of this evaluation is to provide a mechanism by which trending of problem areas can be effectively monitored using the tools of CQI. Based on the trends within any branch, corrective action can be implemented to change processes for improvement. The CSI also provides a method by which implemented corrective action can be evaluated by a simple review of the numbers going up or down and displayed on a run chart.

The client evaluation questionnaire (see Exhibit 4–11) asks five key questions, two of which are broken down by service discipline. The indexing follows these same questions. Scoring is simple: Total number of returned questionnaires divided by total number by category. This simple calculation will allow branch managers and their regional directors to pinpoint specific areas for improvement.

Each month, the indexing scores should be tallied and distributed. Scores should be posted in each branch to allow all employees to be aware of where the office stands in relation to the expectations of management. Examples of indexes are:

1. Staff Performance Index (by discipline)—The expectation should be that the field staff should rank in the 95th percentile.
2. Office Response Index—The expectation is that office staff response to clients should be in the 98th percentile.
3. Client Notification Index (by discipline)—The expectation should be that clients are always notified in advance when there are scheduling problems and when a caregiver can reasonably be expected to be present. One would expect a lower percentile in this index but should set as a minimum the 80th percentile.
4. Client Satisfaction Index—This is a key area to determine whether clients overall were satisfied with services. The expectation is to achieve the 98th percentile.
5. Community Recognition Index—This is another key point to ascertain whether the clients would recommend the agency's services to someone else. The expectation is to achieve the 90th percentile. A sample form is provided in Exhibit 4–11.

If the agency has undertaken the more detailed events-based survey process, it is recommended that the customer satisfaction index be designed using the key drivers of customer satisfaction or key quality characteristics. Using this approach, the index will be able to measure the agency's performance against the most important attributes of customer service. This will be a powerful tool for improvement opportunities.

Exhibit 4-11 Client Evaluation Questionnaire

Your Comments Are Important to Us

As part of our effort to continually improve our services to clients and families, we would appreciate your response to this questionnaire. Your comments will be held in confidence and will assist us in improving our care. We sincerely appreciate your cooperation.

1. How would you rate the overall performance of our staff?

   NURSING:
   Excellent ____
   Good ____
   Fair ____
   Poor ____

   AIDES:
   Excellent ____
   Good ____
   Fair ____
   Poor ____

   THERAPIES:
   Excellent ____
   Good ____
   Fair ____
   Poor ____

   Comments: ____

2. Was the office staff helpful when you called?

   Always ____   Almost Never ____
   Sometimes ____   Never ____
   Comments: ____

3. Did the staff let you know in advance when they would come to your home?

   NURSING:
   Excellent ____
   Good ____
   Fair ____
   Poor ____

   AIDES:
   Excellent ____
   Good ____
   Fair ____
   Poor ____

   THERAPIES:
   Excellent ____
   Good ____
   Fair ____
   Poor ____

   Comments: ____

4. Were you pleased with our services?

   Yes ____   No ____
   Comments: ____

5. Would you recommend our services to someone who needed home care?

   Yes ____   No ____

   Comments: ____
   ____
   ____
   ____
   ____
   ____

   THANK YOU!

   Signed ____

   Date ____

continues

Exhibit 4–11 continued

MISSION STATEMENT

"Enhancing the quality of life through the delivery of compassionate health care at home by skilled professionals continuously striving for excellence"

The above statement is what we tried to accomplish with your care. Please comment on whether or not we accomplished our mission.

We Learn More by Listening Than We Do By Talking.

CLIENT
EVALUATION
QUESTIONNAIRE

Agencies must understand that as the general public's attitudes regarding their expectations continue to mature, customer satisfaction will be a crucial determining factor for success in any community. Most importantly, the public's perception of quality will be based on satisfaction with services rendered.

Agency management should know how quality and value are perceived by its customers. Surveys will answer this and many other questions. Quality is a moving target and as the agency improves, the expectations increase. For this reason, a feedback loop from customers is essential to any quality improvement process. We have discussed many such forms of feedback within this chapter. In the final analysis, however, it is market share that is the real indicator of the quality efforts of an agency. Growth of the agency, or what Deming calls becoming competitive, should be the objective of an agency wishing to remain in business. To this end, it is important that agency administrators understand that technical and relational quality ultimately drive customer satisfaction which, in turn, drive growth and market share. See Figure 4–2.

Technical ability is an internal expectation of management and an external expectation of physicians and other professional sources. Without this expectation being met consistently, referral sources will not continue to refer new patients. Therefore, the agency will not grow. If customers are not consistently satisfied, they will tell their physicians and friends and, again, the result is the same. The agency will not grow over the standard industry growth factor.

The industry growth factor is that percentage by which the home care industry is growing nationally. For example, if nationally, home care grew by 12 percent in 1991 over 1990, then it would be expected that a local agency would have grown by a similar percentage without any marketing effort. Agencies who grew at a significantly lesser pace should do some investigation regarding the community's perception of the agency's quality. Conversely, those agencies who grew at a much higher percentage can feel confident that the community's perception of the agency's quality is good.

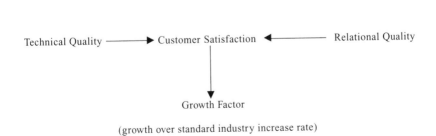

Figure 4–2 Quality Perceptions

CUSTOMER SERVICE STRATEGY

We have discussed obtaining customer feedback regarding the customer's perception of how the agency does business through surveys, questionnaires, and other means. Customer relationship management, however, has another equally important component. It must develop the service strategy employed by the agency to build loyalty in its customers.

There are five customer service strategies agencies should consider:

1. Understanding and use of relational quality
2. Making it easy to do business
3. Treating complaints like gold
4. Balancing recovery with customer life-cycle
5. Implementing lateral service

Understanding and Use of Relational Quality

"Moments of truth" has become a widely accepted term since Jan Carlzon, chief executive officer of SAS Airlines, first used it several years ago. The phrase refers to the proposition that quality is determined by the customer at the point of interaction. Carlzon describes a moment of truth as any point where a customer forms an opinion about the company.

Interactions are events such as scheduling, performing a visit, or just talking to a customer. Each of these interactions provide a basis for customers to judge quality. This type of quality is relational and forms a perception of equal weight to the technical aspects of quality. (See Chapter 2.)

While technical quality, such as sterile technique, is critically important to physicians, relational quality is equally important to the patient. Recently, I observed a focus group of patients and families who all agreed that because of their strong relationship with a local medical office, they could forgive the occasional mistake. These families had confidence that problems would be resolved and they would continue to receive high quality services. Their perception of high quality came directly from the way they were treated. This local office treats their patients like very special people. As a result, when technical quality is occasionally breached, their loyalty continues. The depth of this relationship was not forged overnight, but rather, over a period of time, through numerous transactions.

Conversely, in another situation, a new customer had a trying experience when he had to call an office repeatedly to get some forms delivered to a physician. The office had promised to do so by a certain time and did not. The physician, the patient, and the insurance company all were inconvenienced by this incident.

This new customer's perception of quality is not good and he continues to look for a home care company that can serve his needs.

Relational quality is the art of managing the entire relationship experience. The place to begin is with a "customers come first" attitude. Customers must be the agency's top priority. If every customer were treated like the president of the United States, relational quality would skyrocket and with it, revenues.

In this highly competitive industry, we would do well to remember that if we don't take care of the customer, someone else will.

Making It Easy To Do Business

Today's fast-paced life styles have created a new challenge for all service companies. How to deliver services faster, cheaper, and better than ever. Customers have many choices of service providers; decisions are based on the perception of quality and value. Value is determined from relational and technical quality. Customers have the opportunity to judge value based on a well-established relationship built over time from relational quality perceptions. Customers from insurance company utilization review departments, for example, may never meet or talk to the nurses in a local branch. These customers will form their opinions based on the technical quality of the documentation submitted.

Regardless of the basis for the perception of quality, if agencies are to continue building strong relationships and customer loyalty, they must provide ever-improving value. Home care companies have the opportunity to increase value to all customers by decreasing the cost of doing business. The traditional cost of doing business covers operating expenses and any overhead allocations that may be applicable.

Removing Burdens

A nontraditional aspect to consider in the cost of doing business is to understand the impact on the customer of bureaucratic burdens and delays. Identification of such burdens is not easy, since procedures evolve from internal needs. For example:

- asking customers to research a problem before you can do anything about it
- asking customers to call back for information not readily available
- calling customers back when you didn't get all the information you needed the first time
- asking the customers for forms of verification (such as account numbers) before you can serve them
- all delays are burdens to customers (consider wait times)

Other burdens to customers are errors and omissions on forms. Insurance companies are data driven, they require accurate and complete information before they can make a decision regarding coverage. Any error on a UB–82 could cause a denial while omissions can cause a delay in payments.

Removing these and other potential burdens increases value by making it easier for customers to do business. If customers perceive that services are faster, better, or easier than the competition, revenues and market share will grow!

On the other hand, easing these burdens for customers means increased burdens for the home care agency. Each of the previous examples will create more work for the office unless efficiency is practiced, redundancies removed, and people trained to do the job right the first time. Efficient operations with no burdens on customers creates a value chain that offers faster, cheaper, and better-than-ever services. Providing ever-improving value to customers is a moving target on the fast track to revenue growth, profitability, and increased market share.

Treating Complaints Like Gold

Many health care providers say they hope they never get a customer complaint. Ten lashes with a wet noodle! Agency administrators should hope for lots of complaints. Customer complaints are gifts of gold, and like gold, should be accumulated for the biggest payback on the investment.

How many times have you been disappointed with the service you received but never complained? Instead, you probably won't go back to the business that gave you poor service or didn't treat you well. The disappointed but uncomplaining customer is typical, according to the Technical Assistance Research Programs (TARP), a nationally renowned customer research group.

Customers are motivated to complain only when they care about the relationship with the company or have a strong adverse reaction to some behavior of the company. In either case, the agency should know. TARP's research has revealed that for every customer who does complain, there are 26 others who have the same complaint but will remain silent.[3] These customers simply go elsewhere for their services. If agencies are to continue to increase their market share, they cannot afford to allow any of these silent customers to go to the competition.

Complaints are generally handled very effectively by local offices. However, in multisite agencies, one local office may not know that the cause of a customer complaint in their office may be the same cause of customer complaints in other offices. Because of this lack of shared knowledge, process problems go undiscovered, root causes are never found, and the problem continues. The "gift of gold" given by one customer is not able to "earn interest" as long as the agency only reacts to individual complaints. Agencies should be able to accumulate the gifts of gold in order to proactively address process problems that cut across location and functional barriers. Root causes of problems are systemic in nature and must be addressed from aggregate data.

It is important to note that a complaint management system is not designed to place blame or affix fault. As strange as it may seem, blaming someone is not the best approach, as noted in the discussions of special versus common causes of variation. The belief that problems causing customer complaints come from ineffective processes, not ineffective people, is fundamental to CQI and total quality management (TQM). Employees are merely working within the constraints of the systems and procedures imposed upon them. To correct problems, systems and procedures must be corrected by using the tools of CQI.

When on the "front line" with customers, it is easy to say so-and-so messed up or caused the problem that led to a complaint. While this has been the traditional approach, management should move to a more analytical approach by asking what system, process, or procedure allowed the employee to make the error.

Analyzing a problem by determining which system failed to meet customer expectations and why, will enable agency leadership to address solutions that will have a sustained effect on problem prevention.

While these concepts are new and will take time to fully appreciate, agencies can begin by accepting the gifts of gold from customers with gratitude and understanding of their true value in building a better agency.

Balancing Recovery with Customer Life-Cycle

A plan designed to strengthen customer loyalty is the purpose behind a good recovery strategy. Customer research from TARP has revealed a unique phenomenon: customers who complained and received "above and beyond" recovery are more loyal than customers who have never had a problem.[4]

Occasionally, errors will be made or a problem will occur for a customer. When these things happen, there is an opportunity to exceed expectations by doing something more than is required to satisfy the customer.

For example, I took my car to the dealer to have the mirror repaired, which was supposed to take no more than an hour. I took my laptop computer to do some work while waiting. I was engrossed in my work and did not realize that an hour and a half had gone by. When I inquired as to the status of my car, they had not started the repairs. After a few minutes they understood how unhappy I was with this lack of service. They immediately repaired the mirror (20 minutes) and did not charge me for the service. I was satisfied with the outcome. However, the manager of the service department brought my car around and gave me a certificate for a complete servicing on my car. The certificate had a value of approximately $150. I did not expect this added value in their recovery strategy. But because I got it, I completely forgot my anger and was impressed at how much they wanted to keep my business. They now have a loyal customer.

In another example, I recently held a focus group in Kansas. The hotel used faulty equipment for the videotaping and those observing could neither see nor hear the proceedings. I made my displeasure known and the hotel manager "comped" the charges for the room and the equipment. While this satisfied me enough to continue with plans for the week, I will not be a customer of this hotel in the future. In fact, I strongly recommended that another meeting scheduled for this same hotel be held elsewhere.

The difference between these two examples shows that the dealership cared enough about my future business to take a loss on the current business, while the hotel attempted to minimize their losses. They were not concerned about my future business and as a result, they lost me as a customer.

The reaction of the hotel is typical when something goes wrong. Management attempts to minimize the loss for the one occurrence rather than concentrate on retaining the customer for future business.

Service recovery involves balancing a temporary loss with the life-cycle of customers' business. For example, a managed care customer may have a value to a large home care agency of $200,000 in annual revenue. Over the life-cycle of this customer (estimated at 10 years) the agency may be able to generate approximately $2 million in revenue. Therefore, when a problem occurs, balanced recovery should be thought of not in terms of the visit or the specific problem, but rather, in terms of potentially losing $2 million in revenue.

This balanced perspective on recovery places the emphasis on exceeding rather than merely satisfying the customer's expectations in order to retain the business. This type of recovery strategy will pay back big dividends when used synergistically with other quality improvement initiatives.

Implementing Lateral Service

Lateral service is a concept whose time has come. Today's customer-conscious health care community has accepted that the customer is king once again! Lateral service transforms the organization from one driven by internal policy and procedures to one driven by the desire to satisfy customers. This transformation comes from seeing the company from the customer's viewpoint and acting accordingly.

For example, customers do not see the functional barriers between departments or different locations. Nor do they see a difference between ancillary contractors or PRN personnel and regular employees. Customers see that the agency is one company and they have an expectation that the agency will treat their business the same from location to location or from department to department.

Lateral service enables employees to serve their customers without fear of stepping on toes or ramifications. This concept empowers each employee to satisfy customers' needs whether or not it is within their jurisdiction to do so. If a customer is angry about a problem and contacts the agency, personnel must be empowered to instantly "pacify" him or her. Instant pacification is the art of making customers feel their concerns have been heard and that the problem will be satisfactorily resolved.

In lateral service, the employee who hears a complaint, owns the complaint. This employee must then be responsible for ensuring resolution for the customer. The resolution may take several hours, and may not be resolved by the person who took the call, but the "owner" is responsible for getting back to the customer and following up.

Lateral service is also the ability to anticipate customers' needs. This anticipation of customer needs adds value to the relationship and delights customers. Nurses are especially good at anticipating patients' needs but this concept goes beyond nursing care. It addresses the entire relationship experience. Anticipation is another facet of the good planing and prevention that satisfies customers.

Lateral service empowers the front-line customer contact personnel, including the caregivers, to do whatever it takes to satisfy their customers. Obviously, this statement is meant to imply that satisfaction must occur within the constraints of civil and criminal law. Too often, customers have become angrier because they were forced to repeat their story over and over to different people as they worked their way up to someone who could solve their problem. Lateral service prevents this "customer shuffle" and enables employees to be accountable to the customers they serve.

Each of the foregoing strategies are designed to enhance the relationship experience between the agency and patients, physicians, social workers, and any other customer. Customer service, like all aspects of doing business, requires a plan that follows a prescribed path. Customer-driven quality is a strategic concept that addresses doing business a new way, using the principles and concepts of TQM and CQI.

USING AUDIT TOOLS

With all the audits and surveys and questionnaires, the final analysis of quality will be in the community's perception and continued growth. As an agency's quality improves, new nurses will be more willing to join the agency and stay. Therefore, quality can no longer be perceived as "one of those things nurses do."

Quality is the job of each and every employee, each and every time he or she interfaces with a customer.

NOTES

1. W.E. Deming, *The Quality/Productivity Model* (Japan Management, 1950).

2. L.R. Ericksen, *Nursing Management* (July 1989).

3. TARP, Technical Assistance Research Programs, John Goodman, Executive Director.

4. Speech by John Goodman, Inside America, Making Service Quality Work, Conference of Success Stories in Service Quality, Washington, D.C., 1988.

Chapter 5

National and International Standards

The health care industry has considered itself to be so different for so long that it has become isolated from the mainstream of quality principles. Happily, the Demonstration Project successfully proved that the health care industry can use the tools and techniques of continuous quality improvement (CQI) just as effectively as manufacturing or other industrial businesses. The concepts of CQI can begin to mainstream the home care industry with general business and manufacturing quality principles.

This chapter will explore non-health care national and international standards for quality and their application in the home care environment. It will become apparent that quality with its principles and concepts are universal. Quality by community perception is a process of building a strategic program of customer relationship management. These building "blocks" go from a "commercial" grade of quality up to conformance grade and finally to world-class, where customers are dazzled. An illustration of these ideas can be found in Figure 5–1.

The days of believing the health care industry is different are over. The services provided are different, to be sure, but the fundamental concepts that drive the services are no different from any other service industry. People are the same the world over, and the principles of kindness, fairness, and payment for value are universally applicable.

THE MALCOLM BALDRIGE NATIONAL QUALITY AWARD

The Malcolm Baldrige National Quality Award is an annual award to recognize American companies that excel in quality achievement and quality management. The award has fostered a better partnership between the private sector and the federal government. Robert Mosbacher, the former Secretary of Commerce, said, "This award offers a unique mechanism for cooperation between busi-

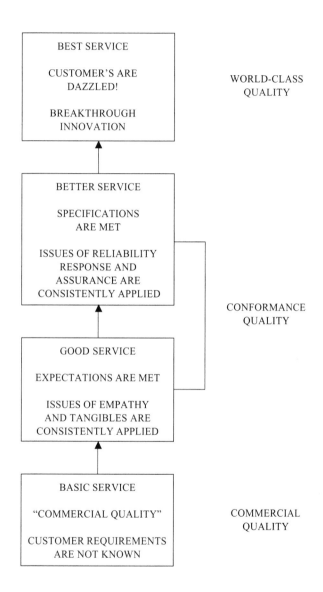

Figure 5–1 Service Blocks to World-Class

ness leaders and quality experts throughout the private sector and government . . ."[1]

The Baldrige was a result of public Law 100–107, signed into law August 20, 1987. Principal support for the program comes from the Foundation for the Malcolm Baldrige National Quality Award, established in 1988. The award is named for Malcolm Baldrige, who served as Secretary of Commerce from 1981 until his death in a rodeo accident in 1987.[2]

The Findings and Purpose of Public Law 100–107, reprinted from the 1990 Award Guidelines, can be found in Exhibit 5–1.

The Baldrige Award has become the de facto standard for quality in America. Internationally, there is a great deal of interest in the Baldrige as industrialized nations clamor to recognize quality as a national priority. The Baldrige Award has become the catalyst for American businesses in recognizing quality as a strategic imperative. The award is given by the president of the United States to the companies that exemplify the highest standards of quality. The award is given in three categories: (1) manufacturing, (2) service, and (3) small business.

As of this writing, the Baldrige Award is limited to for-profit companies. Many home care providers are not-for-profit. However, discussions are now underway to explore the possibility of establishing a new category for health care organizations. Other than the profit status of the corporation, there is nothing in the guidelines that would preclude a home care agency from applying for this prestigious award.

It should be noted that applying for this award for the sake of the trophy is strongly discouraged. The purpose of the award and all it represents is to foster ever-improving quality and value for customers. The guidelines of the Baldrige form a framework for a quality system that has universal application to businesses in any industry. These guidelines are nonprescriptive and offer a basis for a quality system that can propel companies into world-class status. The guidelines from the Baldrige should be seen as a roadmap to follow on a total quality transformation.

Key Concepts of the Baldrige

The award is built upon some key concepts that the reader will recognize from previous chapters in this text. These concepts are:

1. Quality is defined by the customer.
2. Senior managers should create clear quality values (mission) and build these values into the way the company operates.
3. Quality excellence derives from well-designed and well-executed systems and processes.

Exhibit 5–1 The Malcolm Baldrige National Quality Improvement Act of 1987—Public Law 100–107

The Findings and Purposes Section of Public Law 100–107 states that:

1. The leadership of the United States in product and process quality has been challenged strongly (and sometimes successfully) by foreign competition, and our Nation's productivity growth has improved less than our competitors over the last two decades.

2. American business and industry are beginning to understand that poor quality costs companies as much as 20 percent of sales revenues nationally, and that improved quality of goods and services goes hand in hand with improved productivity, lower costs, and increased profitability.

3. Strategic planning for quality and quality improvement programs, through a commitment to excellence in manufacturing and services, are becoming more and more essential to the well-being of our Nation's economy and our ability to compete effectively in the global marketplace.

4. Improved management understanding of the factory floor, worker involvement in quality, and greater emphasis on statistical process control can lead to dramatic improvements in the cost and quality of manufactured products.

5. The concept of quality improvement is directly applicable to small companies as well as large, to service industries as well as manufacturing, and to the public sector as well as private enterprise.

6. In order to be successful, quality improvement programs must be management-led and customer-oriented and this may require fundamental changes in the way companies and agencies do business.

7. Several major industrial nations have successfully coupled rigorous private sector quality audits with national awards giving special recognition to those enterprises the audits identify as the very best.

8. A national quality award program of this kind in the United States would help improve quality and productivity by:

   A. helping to stimulate American companies to improve quality and productivity for the pride of recognition while obtaining a competitive edge through increased profits;

   B. recognizing the achievements of those companies which improve the quality of their goods and services and providing an example to others;

   C. establishing guidelines and criteria that can be used by business, industrial, governmental, and other organizations in evaluating their own quality improvement efforts; and

   D. providing specific guidance for other American organizations that wish to learn how to manage for high quality by making available detailed information on how winning organizations were able to change their cultures and achieve eminence.

Source: The 1990 Malcolm Baldrige National Quality Award Guidelines.

4. Continuous improvement must be a part of the management of all systems and processes.
5. Goals and strategic plans should be developed to achieve quality leadership.
6. Shortening operational and process response time should be a part of the quality improvement effort.
7. Operational decisions need to be based upon facts and data.
8. All employees must be trained and involved in quality activities.
9. Design quality and error prevention should be major elements of the quality system.
10. Companies need to communicate quality requirements to suppliers and contractors and work to evaluate their quality performance.

These ten important concepts come together in the actual award categories discussed below.

Leadership

This category examines how the executives create and sustain clear and visible quality values along with a system to guide all activities of the company toward excellence. Quality leadership displayed in the community and how the company integrates its public responsibilities with its quality values and practices are also examined.

Goal setting, planning, review of quality achievement, and recognizing employees for quality performance are methods management can use to reinforce the quality values of the company. The senior executive's personal involvement in developing and maintaining an environment for quality excellence is the strongest element in this category. As discussed previously, continuous quality improvement must be management-led.

Another key quality characteristic under this category is how management integrates the quality values into daily operational leadership and how the management of all units reinforces these values.

Information and Analysis

This category examines the scope, validity, use, and management of data supporting the company's quality management system. Also examined is the adequacy of the data, information, or analysis to support a responsive, prevention-based approach to quality and customer satisfaction.

Meeting quality improvement goals requires that actions in setting, controlling, and changing processes be based on reliable data. A major consideration relating to data and analysis in connection with quality system development for continuous improvement involves the creation and use of performance indicators. These indicators should be measurable characteristics used to evaluate performance. The indicators should be selected based on those attributes that link to customer requirements (added value) or link to customer satisfaction or operational effectiveness and efficiency. Key quality characteristics are excellent indicators when used to measure performance. Outcome indicators can also be used in this category.

A system of indicators developed in this manner represents an objective basis for aligning all activities of the company toward well-defined goals. With the process of continuous improvement, these goals would change as the data indicated. In other words, as goals are met and customers come to expect that level of performance, the "bar" goes up. When a performance indicator is precedent-setting, such as the 10:30 A.M. guaranteed delivery by Federal Express, the competition is compelled to at least match the performance in order to stay competitive.

Another objective under this category is the ability of the company to benchmark. This practice is one home care providers have long used and is simply the sharing of information between companies. In this context, benchmarking is done for the purpose of making comparisons on quality-related issues in order to emulate the best of the best both within the industry and outside of it. A detailed discussion of benchmarking appears in the Quality and Operational Results category. It is important to note at this point that benchmarking is the identification of practices that can be emulated within the home care industry. It is not limited to companies within this industry. For example, a home care company may want to benchmark Toyota Corporation for its employee suggestion program, AT&T Universal Card Center for its inquiry system, the Ritz Carlton for their customer service program, and Motorola for their six sigma quality. If an agency limits its benchmarking program to only those companies within the home care industry, best in industry may be possible but not best in class or world-class.

Strategic Quality Planning

This category addresses the company's planning process for achieving (or retaining) quality leadership and how the company integrates quality improvement planning into the overall business plan. The company's short- and long-range plans are reviewed to validate the achievement and retention of quality leadership.

The company's process for strategic planning is reviewed in relationship to the issues of quality and customer satisfaction. The focus of the review is on the process of planning and goal setting, and integration of the quality plans with the agency's overall business plans. Home care agencies have traditionally developed their quality plans outside the scope of business planning. In fact, the Joint Commission has never encouraged any other practice. Today, however, quality planning cannot be segregated from business planning. Total quality dictates that quality is the manner in which business is done. The alignment concepts of total quality management (TQM) necessitate that the strategic quality plan be an all-encompassing document that covers all business planning activities of the agency.

Human Resource Development and Management

This category is one of the most important in the Malcolm Baldrige. The category examines the effectiveness of the company's efforts to develop and realize the full potential of the work force and to maintain an environment conducive to full participation, quality leadership, and personal and organizational growth.

Meeting the company's quality objectives requires a fully committed, well-trained group of employees that is stimulated to work for continuous improvements. Reward and recognition systems should reinforce participation in the quality systems. Additionally, recognition programs should emphasize achievement of quality objectives. Factors that bear upon the safety, health, well-being, and morale of employees need to be a part of the CQI system. The methods available for employee participation in the quality program will be examined, as will their contribution toward quality goals. Trends and current levels of participation will be reviewed.

Employees should receive training in basic quality skills of CQI and statistical process control as it relates to their job and to understanding and solving quality-related problems and improving processes. How the company decides on what kind of quality training and education is made available will be reviewed. A summary of all employee training by type and job classification will be assessed.

This is the category that assures alignment with all quality plans and goals. The real proof of a quality system is when the employees know it, run it, improve it, and are rewarded for it. Another proof of alignment in this category is if the actual practices at all levels of the organization reflect the plans for quality improvement and exceed customer expectations. The real test of "walk-the-talk" is validated within this category.

Management of Process Quality

This category examines the systematic approaches used for assuring quality based upon process design and control. This includes the process of assuring quality for contracted services or procured supplies, equipment, and other administrative services. The company will be asked to describe the quality of services furnished by outside contractors or suppliers and how those services are assured, assessed, and improved. Also examined is the integration of process control and improvement with the quality program.

The review will include how new services are designed and introduced and how processes are designed to meet key service quality characteristics. What type of processes the company uses to produce its services and how these processes are controlled are key variables under this category. Additionally, questions relating to company service improvement will be examined.

The assessment process for the quality of processes, systems, practices, and services will be examined in detail. Documentation requirements for the purpose of transferring and retaining knowledge to support the quality system must be accessible, adequate, and reliable. The company will be asked to summarize process quality, quality assessment, and quality improvement activities for business processes and other support services.

Achieving the highest levels of quality and competitiveness will require a well-defined and well-executed approach to CQI of all processes, departments, and operations. Improvements may be of several types:

- enhancing value to the customer through improved service attributes
- reducing errors and defects
- improving responsiveness and cycle-time performance
- improving efficiency and effectiveness in the use of all resources

To meet these requirements, the continuous improvement process must contain regular intervals of planning, execution, and evaluation. It must be accomplished based on quantitative, objective data.

The reduction of cycle time and increased responsiveness are gaining momentum in the competitive environment. Fast response time itself is a major competitive advantage as customers' demands for better and faster continue to increase. Reduction in turnaround times and lead times, as well as rapid response to customers, can only occur when quality systems and processes are designed to meet both quality and response goals. This requires that all designs, objectives, and activities include measurements and monitoring of response times, then actively seek to improve those measures. Major improvements in turnaround times can be achieved only when processes are simplified and shortened. Such changes are generally accompanied by simultaneous improvements in output quality. Hence, it is very beneficial to consider response time and quality together. Again, this is the quality–productivity connection, discussed in the Deming model. This issue will be further explored in Chapter 6.

Quality and Operational Results

This category examines quality levels and quality improvements based upon objective measures derived from analysis of customer requirements and expectations and from analysis of business operations. Companies' quality levels are compared against each other using the key quality characteristics and the established goals of the company. Also reviewed are the company's results in quality and performance in comparison to its competition.

Benchmaking quality levels is a major issue under this category. Companies should compare themselves with their own competition and then compare themselves to known world-class companies (not necessarily in the same industry). Summaries of trends from benchmarking will be required. Also required will be summations of quality trends and current quality levels in business processes, operations, and all support services. The same information will be applicable to the service contractors.

This category will confirm the alignment sought in other categories. In other words, results would be necessary to show how the agency performed against key quality characteristics identified from customer research. Trend data would need to be presented to show that the agency has significantly improved over time and that quality levels continue to improve for all key indicators of quality and performance. This category is almost always presented in graphic form.

Customer Satisfaction and Relationship Management

By far the largest and most important category in the Baldrige Award is customer satisfaction, which is reflective of the first concept of quality—quality is determined by the customer. This category examines the company's knowledge of the customer, its basis for that knowledge, and its ability to meet the customer's expectations. The customer service systems in place are examined, as well as current levels and trends in customer satisfaction.

How the company determines current and future customer requirements and expectations will be reviewed. How the company manages its relationship with its customers and how it uses information gained from customers to improve services will be looked at in detail. The management of customer relationships is viewed from the perspective of the management practices that enhance customer relationships. Company standards governing the interaction between customers and employees will be examined, including how those standards were set, and subsequently, how they are modified (based on applicable data).

The company's commitment to customers will be reviewed in light of the company's own explicit and implicit promises underlying the services it provides. How the company handles and resolves complaints and uses complaint information for quality improvement and preventing recurrence of problems also will be examined.

The description of methods for determining customer satisfaction and how that information is used in quality improvement will be addressed. Additionally, summaries will be requested identifying trends in customer satisfaction and in indicators of adverse customer responses. These trends will be benchmarked against industry competition.

The preceding information has been excerpted from the Malcolm Baldrige National Quality Award Guidelines, the symbol for which is found in Figure 5–2. The guidelines have been included in this book to illustrate the applicability of industry quality standards to home care. Additionally, it is important to reflect on the lack of inspection techniques in these standards. As this book points out, quality must be built into the service, not inspected in. As discussed previously in this text, however, this does not mean that inspection (traditional quality assurance [QA]) should not occur. It does mean that

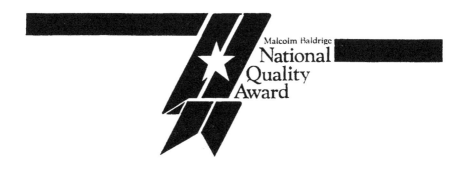

"The improvement of quality in products and the improvement of quality in service — these are national priorities as never before."

George Bush

Figure 5–2 Malcolm Baldrige National Quality Award Symbol. *Source:* The 1991 Malcolm Baldrige National Quality Award Guidelines (front cover).

inspection should not be used as the only means of assuring quality. The category for management of process quality does have a section that deals with how the agency assures quality. It would be expected that agencies would use statistical means to sustain and continually improve all quality outcomes.

The other point worthy of reflection is the constant reinforcement of the need for decisions to be based on quantifiable, objective data and the need for these data to be used as a basis for continuous quality improvement.

This point reflects the concept that organizations should manage by fact, not intuition.

A final point that should be mentioned is the overwhelming reliance on customers for the determination of quality. This customer-driven approach is a new concept to the health care industry, but one that can revolutionize the manner in which health care is rendered in this country.

INTERNATIONAL STANDARDS ORGANIZATION 9000–9004 SERIES OF QUALITY MANAGEMENT AND QUALITY ASSURANCE STANDARDS

The purpose of having international standards agreed to by the major industrial nations of the world is to bring operational definition to quality standards that have the same meaning and interpretation for all. The International Standards Organization (ISO) developed the Series 9000–9004 in an effort to make world trade more compatible. For example, if you buy a VCR in England, it will be basically the same product you would buy in the United States and vice versa. Compatibility of goods and services enhances international trade and understanding. This compatibility is similar to the standardization of processes.

The computer industry is one of the last to adopt the standardization for quality theme. For the first time computer companies are beginning to standardize software so that it can be used on any computer, and the hardware requirements are beginning to allow for the "marrying" of different products. It will be wonderful when users no longer have to worry about what software is compatible with their home personal computer.

Think how difficult the world would be without standardization. Almost everything in our lives has been standardized, which has added to our quality of life and overall satisfaction. Suppose, for example, that I go to the video store for a movie and the video cassette doesn't fit the VCR. Suppose I go to the grocery store for lightbulbs and find they won't fit. Suppose my heater breaks down and there are no parts that fit. We have so internalized this concept of standardization that we have come to regard it as a subliminal expectation.

The ISO 9000–9004 Series attempts to standardize the quality discipline into operational definitions that all companies doing business anywhere in the world can understand and comply with. These standards were developed for manufacturing and other industry; yet, as we have seen from the standards of the Baldrige Award, quality is a universal language.

The international standards were "Americanized" by the American Society for Quality Control, which participated in their development. The following summations of the ISO Standards were taken from the American National Standards (the American equivalent of ISO Standards).

Quality Management and Quality Assurance Standards[3]

A principal factor in the performance of an organization is the quality of its products and services. There is a world-wide trend toward more stringent customer expectations with regard to quality. Accompanying this trend has been a growing realization that continual improvements in quality are often necessary to achieve and sustain good economic performance.

These standards recommend that a quality policy be adopted by all companies that defines the overall quality intentions and directions as expressed and deployed by top management. The standards specifically give the responsibility for quality management to senior leaders.

The standards specify that unless given requirements fully reflect the needs of the user, quality assurance cannot be complete. For effectiveness, quality assurance requires continuing evaluation of factors that affect the adequacy of the design or specification for end use.

An organization should seek to accomplish the following three objectives with regard to the quality policy:

1. The organization should achieve and sustain the quality of service so as to meet continually the purchaser's stated or implied needs.
2. The organization should provide confidence to its own management that the intended quality is being achieved and sustained.
3. The organization should provide confidence to the purchaser that the intended quality is being or will be achieved in the delivered service.

The quality system elements should be documented and demonstrable in a manner consistent with requirements of the customer. In this regard, the standards identify criteria for the demonstration of the quality system:

- adequacy of the quality system
- capability to achieve service conformity with specified requirements

Documentation may include manuals, descriptions of processes, operational definition, quality system auditing reports, and statistical methods reports.

Quality Systems—Model for Quality Assurance[4]

The company shall identify verification requirements and provide adequate resources to carry out this function, including assigning trained personnel for verification activities. Such activities shall include inspection, monitoring of process and service, and audits of the quality system and shall be carried out by personnel *independent* of those having responsibility for the work being performed.

The company shall establish and maintain a documented quality system as a means of ensuring that the service conforms to specified requirements. Documentation shall include:

1. quality system operational definitions
2. effective implementation of documented quality system procedures and instructions
3. preparation of quality plans and a quality manual
4. identification of controls, processes, and skills that may be needed to achieve the required quality
5. updating of all controls and processes as needed
6. clarification of standards of acceptability for all features and requirements, including any that may contain a subjective element
7. compatibility of the documentation to the process design and procedures

The company shall ensure that services conform to specified requirements. For those services furnished by subcontractors, the company shall make selections based on the contractor's ability to meet the specified requirements. Appropriate records shall be maintained on all acceptable subcontractors.

The company shall establish, document, and maintain procedures for the following:

1. investigating the cause of nonconformity and the corrective action needed to prevent future occurrence
2. analyzing all processes, operations, complaints, etc. to detect and eliminate potential causes for nonconformity
3. initiating preventive actions to deal with problems to a level corresponding to the risks encountered
4. applying controls to ensure that corrective actions are taken and that they are effective
5. implementing and documenting changes in procedures and processes resulting from corrective action

The company shall carry out a comprehensive system of planned and documented internal quality audits to verify whether quality activities comply with planned arrangements and to determine the effectiveness of the quality system. Management shall take timely and appropriate action to correct and prevent deficiencies. The company shall establish procedures for identifying adequate statistical techniques required for verifying the acceptability of process capability.

Final Inspection and Testing[5]

The company shall establish and maintain an effective quality system for inspection and testing. This shall include documentation of procedures for final inspection, including standards for job classifications and standards for quality records. The company shall carry out final inspection in accordance with documented procedures. The inspection shall include a verification of acceptable results for the purpose of verifying that requirements have been met.

Quality Management and Quality System Elements[6]

In order to meet its objectives, the company should organize itself in such a way that the technical, administrative, and human factors affecting the quality of services will be under control. The company's quality management system has two interrelated aspects:

1. The company's needs and interests: For the company, there is a business need to attain and maintain the desired quality at an optimum cost; the fulfillment of this quality aspect is related to the planned and efficient utilization of the technological, human, and other resources available to the company.
2. The customer's needs and expectations: For the customer, there is a need for confidence in the ability of the company to deliver the desired quality consistently.

Each of these two aspects of the quality management system requires objective evidence in the form of data concerning the quality of the system and the quality of the company's services.

Risk, cost, and benefit considerations have great importance to both the company and the customer. These considerations are:

1. Risk considerations:
   - Consideration must be given to company risks related to deficient services, which lead to loss of image or reputation, loss of market

share, complaints, claims, liability, and waste of human and financial resources.
- Equal consideration must be given to risks for customers, such as those pertaining to the safety and welfare of patients, dissatisfaction with services, lack of availability, and loss of confidence.
2. Cost considerations:
- For companies, consideration must be given to costs due to marketing, process deficiencies, rework, reprocessing, etc.
- For the customer, consideration must be given to safety and downtime.
3. Benefit considerations:
- For the company, consideration must be given to increased profitability and market share.
- For the customer, consideration must be given to improved safety and health, increased satisfaction, and growth in confidence.

An effective quality management system should be designed to satisfy customer needs and expectations while serving to protect the company's interests. A well-structured quality system is a valuable management resource in the optimization and control of quality in relation to risk, cost, and benefit considerations. The emphasis of the quality system should be on problem prevention rather than dependence on detection after occurrence.

The impact of quality upon the profit and loss statement can be highly significant, particularly in the long term. It is, therefore, important that the effectiveness of the system be measured in a businesslike manner. The main objective of quality cost reporting is to provide a means for evaluating effectiveness and establishing the basis for the internal improvement program.

It should be common practice to identify and measure quality costs as those costs directed at achieving appropriate levels of quality and resultant costs from inadequate control. These costs could include:

- prevention
- inspection
- internal failure (failure prior to delivery)
- external failure (failure after delivery)
- costs associated with proof of quality required by customers

These quality costs should be regularly reported to and monitored by management and be related to other costs (ratio) measures to allow management to:

1. evaluate the adequacy and effectiveness of the quality management system
2. identify additional areas requiring attention
3. establish quality and cost objectives

The company should establish and maintain an information and monitoring system of customer feedback on a continuous basis. All data gathered should be analyzed, collated, interpreted, and communicated in accordance with written procedure.

If a problem is identified, the root cause should be determined before preventive measures are planned. Often the root cause is not obvious, thus requiring careful analysis of the service specification that produced the problem. Additionally, all related processes, operations, quality records, and customer complaints should be reviewed to determine the root cause. Statistical methods are useful in determining root cause and in problem analysis. It should be emphasized that statistical methods are an important element in the quality system and should be used throughout the company.

About now, this should all be starting to sound familiar. Isn't it amazing that the home care industry has so much in common with other businesses and industries the world over?

NOTES

1. *Malcolm Baldrige National Quality Award Guidelines*, 1991.

2. D.M. Berwick, A.B. Godfrey, J. Roessner, *A Report on the National Demonstration Project on Quality Improvement in Health Care, Curing Health Care* (San Fancisco: Jossey-Bass, 1991).

3. *American National Standard, Quality Management and Quality Assurance Standards—Guidelines for Selection and Use* (American Society for Quality Control, 1987).

4. *American National Standard, Quality Systems—Model for Quality Assurance in Design/Development, Production, Installation and Servicing* (American Society for Quality Control, 1987).

5. *American National Standard, Quality Systems—Model for Quality Assurance in Final Inspection and Test* (American Society for Quality Control, 1987).

6. *American National Standard, Quality Management and Quality System Elements—Guidelines* (American Society for Quality Control, 1987).

Chapter 6
The Quality–Productivity Connection

The Deming model for quality and productivity discussed in Chapter 1 detailed the relationship between quality and productivity. This connection has to do with an issue we have touched on briefly: cycle time. As mentioned in Chapter 2, cycle time will be the top competitive advantage of the 1990s. Fast response, or cycle time, is a customer satisfier and often creates a major service differentiator among competitive organizations. For example, if your agency is the only one that can consistently send a nurse to the bedside of a patient within two hours of hospital discharge, you have created a service differentiator in the community. If this is an important service attribute, the agency that consistently meets this requirement will get the referrals.

Quality enables cycle-time reduction. The better the quality, the faster the response time. Tom Peters, a management consultant, tells of an insurance company that reduced its policy processing time from 17 days to 22 minutes. This dramatic reduction in time was a result of a process reengineering project that simplified the process of issuing a policy. Additionally, this company was able to consolidate approvals into the front-line employee, with parameters clearly spelled out in operational definition.

This example highlights the fact that cycle time drives quality improvement. As your customers require faster, cheaper, and better-than-ever services, home care providers will be forced to rethink the way they do business. This process forces agencies to review all delay time usually caused by pass-offs or approvals of another person. Another major contributor to delay time is overly complicated processes. Regarding the cost of doing business, wait time is a waste cost to customers and the agency. All delays should be avoided.

As discussed in Chapter 2, in order to improve cycle time, the emphasis should be on the design of the process or procedure rather than on the individual employee. This breaks tradition with the old industrial engineering model that did time studies on employees to improve efficiency. While this model is still useful, it should be used only to set parameters of performance and then only as a basis for improvement thereafter.

In addition to emphasizing process design or redesign, agency administrators should pay close attention to prevention of error and defect as a means of improving response time. Also, consideration should be given to the organization of the agency, communications within it, and the flexibility of staff in problem solving. Staff flexibility refers to the extent to which the staff have been empowered to act on behalf of their customers.

Cycle time should be measured in the aggregate and for each of the process steps in order to determine opportunities for improvement. In fact, service-related cycle-time issues will likely become key quality characteristics as identified from customer-based research. When cycle time becomes a standard, consistency is the key to the ability to offer a service guarantee on this basis.

All of the concepts, principles, and theories discussed in this book will require a paradigm shift in everyone within the agency to make quality improvement a reality. A paradigm serves as the framework for a thought process. It acts as a gatekeeper to the thought process by filtering information based on the totality of one's experiences. This filtering can actually translate information based on one's current knowledge and experience. For example, the country has been going through a paradigm shift in the way we take care of ourselves. Years ago, it was socially acceptable to smoke in a room with others without consideration for their feelings. It was an acceptable way of life to eat foods high in cholesterol, sugar, and salt. Today all that has changed.

With repetition, paradigms will shift into the acceptance of new tools, techniques, and methods. As acceptance grows and these methods are consistently applied, productivity will significantly improve.

How many times have you heard someone say, "If you did it right the first time, you wouldn't have to do it over"? As children, we heard this statement many times. We learned every behavior we practice today by the same process—repetition. The more we do something, the better we get at it until it becomes second nature. This is the process of acquiring and maintaining overlearned skills.

The process of developing overlearned skills can be applied to issues regarding improved quality. For example, a nurse can look at a patient and know if trouble is imminent by automatically looking for signs and symptoms. The assessment skills learned and routinely practiced every day make this process an overlearned skill. The nurse is not consciously thinking about the process of assessment while observing the patient.

THE THOUGHT PROCESS

For our purpose we will look at two areas of the thought process:

1. conscious thought
   - perception
   - association
   - evaluation
   - decision
2. subconscious thought
   - stores information
   - handles overlearned skills

Conscious Thought

When quality standards are introduced into an agency for the first time, nurses must consciously think through the process. All the steps of conscious thought must be gone through.

Perception

The nurse or other staff member must perceive the standards as being realistic, attainable, and in keeping with generally accepted nursing practice. This perception must be the individual's perception, not just the perception of management. If the nurse's perception is that the standard is too high or otherwise not realistic, the chances of that nurse "buying in" are remote. Without a buy-in by the staff, the goals of quality improvement will not be realized.

Association

The employee must be able to make a direct association between the quality standards and improved patient care. This association must be internalized by the staff who will ultimately associate the standards with improved patient outcomes. Again, the nurse or other staff member must buy in to this association; it cannot be imposed by management.

Evaluation

The employee must be able to evaluate the perceived results as worthwhile and beneficial to his or her individual practice. The anticipation is that the employee should be able to draw a closer connection between theoretical knowledge and professional practice by utilizing these standards. If this connection occurs, the employee will evaluate the quality improvement process as necessary to the specific care that he or she will be rendering.

Decision

The decision to act in a specific manner will be determined as a result of each of the previously mentioned steps. The employee must perceive that the quality standards are good, must associate the standards with improved practice, and must evaluate the standards as aids to improved performance. If all of these processes take place, the employee's decision will be to meet the standards and behave accordingly.

Subconscious Thought

It will be the responsibility of management to introduce the standards in a positive way and to allow input from the field staff who must ultimately "own" the standards. In fact, the staff should be involved in the development of the standards. Once the staff has accepted the standards and begun the process of application, then repetition will eventually turn the standards into behaviors that will become overlearned skills. It is important to remember that during the process of employees applying new standards, close supervision and monitoring will be necessary. If a procedure or skill is incorrectly applied and becomes overlearned, it is extremely difficult to change the behavior. Supervisors must ensure that each employee is applying the standard correctly *before* it becomes an overlearned skill.

During the process of initiating quality standards, it is essential that the supervisor focus on the desired behavioral expectations. Emphasis should not be placed on inappropriate behavior. Managers can predict or perpetuate performance with the words used. Every word, action, and deed should be given in a positive manner.

Supervisors should be aware that reflective thinking comes from the words employees hear, which create pictures in the mind, which create the feelings one gets. It is the resulting feeling that will act as the catalyst to change behaviors. Supervisors should want to instill in the staff a feeling of positive change. An old Chinese proverb says, "The mind is like a parachute—it works better when opened."

MOTIVATIONAL THEORIES

Motivational theories attempt to explain what it takes to get people to behave in a certain manner. All managers have worked through these at some time in their career. A brief review will be provided as a refresher.

Maslow's Hierarchy

A very popular theory of motivation that bases all behaviors on individual needs was articulated by Maslow. The Maslow theory of hierarchy of needs postulates that only those needs that have not been met will motivate behavior. Maslow believed that a person's needs are arranged in a hierarchy of importance.[1]

1. physiological needs—basic survival needs (i.e., food, water, and shelter)
2. safety and security needs—the need for protection from harm
3. affection and social activity needs—needs for association, friendship
4. esteem and status needs—needs for recognition and appreciation
5. self-actualization needs—the need for self-fulfillment or to reach one's potential

Figure 6–1 illustrates the Maslow Hierarchy of needs.

Learned-Need Theory

McClelland, like Maslow, believed that behavior was motivated by needs. He grouped the identified needs into only three categories: achievement, power, and affiliation.[2] McClelland's subsequent research with business managers led him to believe that of the three need categories, power was the most important for this group of people. If the McClelland theory is to be believed, power will become a major obstacle to overcome in the transformation to continuous quality improvement. Continuous quality improvement is about empowerment, sharing of power, and breaking down the traditional barriers between the managers and the workers.

Two-Factor Theory

The two-factor theory is based on employees either being satisfied or dissatisfied. Motivation was divided into two categories by Frederick Herzberg and his associates.

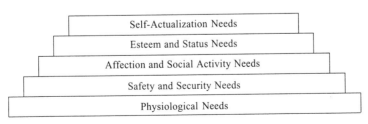

Figure 6–1 Maslow's Hierarchy of Needs. *Source:* Reprinted from Maslow, A.H., A Theory of Human Motivation, in *Psychological Review,* July 1943, pp. 370–396.

1. motivators—increase job satisfaction and performance
2. hygiene factors—do not contribute to motivation but their absence leads to dissatisfaction, i.e., demotivators

This theory also forms the basis for customer satisfaction. Customers may not articulate certain issues because they have come to expect that these things will be a routine part of service delivery. However, their absence will lead to dissatisfaction if not met. For example, customers do not articulate that they want the caregiver to have clean hands. When the caregiver's hands are clean, it does not add to satisfaction. If the caregiver's hands are dirty, however, the customer will be dissatisfied.

Exhibit 6–1 illustrates Herzberg's theory.

Expectancy Theory

Vroom theorized that motivation comes from the results that one believes will come from certain behavior (for example, the expectation that if you work hard you will get promoted).[3]

Porter and Lawler[4] expanded on the original Vroom theory and acknowledged the relationship between rewards and performance. Porter and Lawler's model suggested that performance causes satisfaction rather than the Vroom theory that satisfaction causes performance.

In either event, the experts agree that there is a relationship between rewards and performance. This relationship gives rise to the performance-based evaluation, performance-based job description, performance-based standards, etc.

The expectancy theories pose a significant challenge to the managers of home care agencies with a desire to be quality driven. Can the industry fashion rewards

---

Exhibit 6–1 Two-Factor Theory

Motivators	Hygiene Factors (Demotivators)
Achievement	Policy/Administration
Recognition	Supervision
Satisfactory Work	Salary
Responsibility	Interpersonal Relations
Advancement	Working Conditions

Source: Herzberg, F., *Work and the Nature of Man,* World Publishing, 1966.

(pay raises, promotions, bonuses, etc.) based on quality outcomes at every level of the operation? Continuous quality improvement will move the industry in this direction. The theories agree on one issue: Employees motivate themselves if the environment is right. The challenge for managers is to create the environment within which people can motivate themselves.

PRODUCTIVITY

Now that the thought process and motivational theory have been reviewed, let us turn our attention to the specifics of productivity:

$$\text{Productivity} = \frac{\text{output}}{\text{input}}$$

This formula can be translated many ways, but an example is that net revenue divided by the total cost of operating will equal the productivity factor, or a percentage of net profit. Many would argue that profit has no place in a discussion on quality. However, making a profit is like breathing; if you don't do it, you die. Whether the agency is nonprofit, proprietary, free-standing, or hospital based, every agency must make a profit to stay in business. Profits also go toward supporting the quality improvement activities necessary to achieve optimum results for patient care.

The productivity of an agency or individual will be a determining factor in quality. For example, if it takes a nurse an hour to insert a Foley catheter, it is likely there was no quality involved. Some nurses have made the assumption that the more time taken, the better the quality. Not so—the reverse is almost always true. A nurse who says he or she can only make three visits per day because he or she is rendering quality care is being neither realistic nor truthful. Inefficiency is not synonymous with quality nor should any manager accept it as such. Cost considerations are playing an increasingly important role in home care with the growth of managed care and prospective payment looming on the horizon. The efficient use of health care resources has become an ethical issue that must be addressed aggressively. Quality care results from consistent conformance to the customer's expectations and requirements, delivered in an efficient manner. The customer is anyone to whom you pass work and is always right. Therefore, the customer can be a patient, client, physician, supervisor, government official, another employee, etc. Quality is synonymous with efficiency and should always be viewed from a time-saving perspective. In other words, it takes less time for a trained, knowledgeable person to do a job than an untrained person. Therefore, it costs less for a well-trained person to do a job than an untrained person. "Well done is better than well said," was a truism of Benjamin Franklin that is still valid today. It costs less to do a job right the first time than to go back to do it over. It also takes less time. The better the quality, the less time the process will take. Productivity ratios of a staff member must be closely monitored to establish patterns of practice. In a certified agency, a ratio of between 1.0 to 1.6 employee hours to visits may be acceptable for a nurse depending on driving time and distance. This ratio considers the number of hours worked divided by the number of visits made:

$$\text{Productivity ratio} = \frac{\text{hours}}{\text{visits}}$$

This ratio is based on averages of all clients and all hours worked by discipline and takes into consideration in-home time, drive time, documentation time, telephone time, and other administrative time. Every employee should know the cost of wasted or unproductive time. This cost is money taken away from patient care and stockholders. Professionals can ill afford to waste money in the health care environment when costs are constantly rising and cost containment is the norm.

Time Study

In order to determine the current productivity ratio of the agency, a time study should be performed. It is important to remember that data make the difference between fact and opinion. Productivity ratios should never be set without the data to support them.

A time study should delineate three separate issues:

1. driving time—use actual odometer readings for mileage
2. in-home time—use actual arrival and departure times
3. administrative time—count all other paid time (including paid time off)

The time study should be done for a period of at least four consecutive weeks by every member of the field staff. It is suggested that the base month (for data gathering) be one in which there are no holidays. If a month where holidays occur cannot be avoided, remove any holiday from the sample.

The following suggested study methodology may be useful:

1. Give an inservice to all caregivers on the purpose of the time study. It is suggested that management be creative in dealing with staff on this issue. Some will consider this type of study a threat to their individual practice and will seek to undermine the concept. It will be important for the staff to understand that exact times must be recorded for accuracy. Rounded times should not be accepted.

2. Have all employees and contractors fill out the time study for a period of one month. Each week's time sheet should be turned in at the end of the work week.

3. Separate the first week's time sheets by discipline and specialty if applicable. For example, all home health aides, physical therapists, and registered nurses will be grouped by discipline. If the agency is active in specialty services such as pediatrics or infusion therapy, these should also be segmented. (*Note:* Separate the registered nurses [RNs] from the licensed practical nurses [LPNs] since their job functions are different.)

4. Average each category of time by discipline and specialty. During this first review, careful scrutiny should be given to the accuracy of the completed time sheet. Do not accept any time sheet that has the times rounded. Reinforce the original instructions.

5. Segment and average every week as the time sheets come in, ensuring that no time sheet is used that has rounded times in any category.

6. At the end of the test period, segment and average all disciplines and specialties into an overall productivity factor for each of the three categories.

7. Add all three categories together by discipline and specialty to get the total productivity factor for each service.

8. Separately sample weekend on-call by discipline.

9. Review results with the staff, and get input for process changes.

It is easier and less time consuming to take the total hours worked and divide by the total visits performed by discipline for the test month. This simple calculation does not require any time study or involvement from the staff. It is not recommended for use in setting the productivity ratios, however, because of its all-inclusive nature. For example, using the shortcut method will not allow agency managers to know where the problem areas are nor will it assist the agency to improve any process that may be contributing to a lack of optimum performance. The time study will prove invaluable to managers who have a desire to improve productivity, not by making caregivers work harder, but by improving processes that could be causing a lack of performance. Exhibit 6–2 illustrates this calculation.

The manager has the opportunity to review these data and act accordingly. For example, assume the manager believed too much time was being spent on administration and the staff concurred. This would be an excellent opportunity to utilize some of the tools of continuous quality improvement (CQI) previously discussed. All the processes that contribute to the necessity of spending an average of 50 minutes on administrative duties per visit would have

Exhibit 6–2 Calculating Results of RN Time Study

```
Driving Time .......................................... 35 minutes per visit
In-Home Time ......................................... 20 minutes per visit
Administrative Time ................................... 50 minutes per visit
Total Time ........................................ 105 minutes = 1.75 hours
Productivity Factor ................................... 1.8 = 22 visits/week
```

to be reviewed by an improvement task team to find ways to reduce this burden. In this case, the processes that would require review would include:

- case conferencing
- documentation
- coordination
- chart review
- scheduling
- supplies

These processes, not the individual nurses, are the barriers to decreasing administrative time. An example of a time study form is shown in Exhibit 6–3.

KEYS TO EXCELLENCE

The quality–productivity connection is one that can produce that for which we all strive—excellence in quality service. Process is the key to excellence just as it is the key to quality.

Components of Excellence

Four components contribute to the achievement of excellence: destiny, future, tools, and skills. Figure 6–2 illustrates these components.

Destiny

Contrary to what some people believe, destiny is not a matter of chance; rather, it is a matter of choice. The selection criteria used will determine the destiny. There are three types of people: the "cans," the "can'ts," and the "won'ts." If you think you can, you can. If you think you can't, you won't. The "cans" are the people who control their destiny and the ones who should be placed in charge of quality improvement. Every person controls his or her destiny through the subconscious. The goals that are internalized will direct the subconscious into appropriate action toward the desired outcome.

Exhibit 6–3 Time Study

```
WEEK _____        NAME _____
DISCIPLINE _____      SPECIALTY _____

*********************************************************************
DAY _____
                                    DEPARTURE
TO: _____  ODOMETER _____  TIME _____
                                    ARRIVAL
                  ODOMETER _____  TIME _____
                                    DEPARTURE
                                    TIME _____
                                    ARRIVAL
TO: _____  ODOMETER _____  TIME _____
                                    DEPARTURE
                                    TIME _____
                                    ARRIVAL
TO: _____  ODOMETER _____  TIME _____
                                    DEPARTURE
                                    TIME _____
                                    ARRIVAL
TO: _____  ODOMETER _____  TIME _____
                                    DEPARTURE
                                    TIME _____
                                    ARRIVAL
TO: _____  ODOMETER _____  TIME _____
                                    DEPARTURE
                                    TIME _____
                                    ARRIVAL
TO: _____  ODOMETER _____  TIME _____
                                    DEPARTURE
                                    TIME _____
                                    ARRIVAL
TO: _____  ODOMETER _____  TIME _____
                                    DEPARTURE
                                    TIME _____

*********************************************************************

                  TOTAL
TOTAL VISITS ____ MILES _____
                  TOTAL             TOTAL
                  DRIVING           IN-HOME
                  TIME _____  TIME _____
                  TOTAL             TOTAL
                  TIME              ADMINISTRATIVE
                  WORKED _____  TIME _____
```

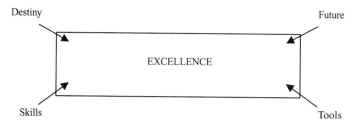

Figure 6–2 Attaining Excellence

Future

If you are not prepared to impose your terms on life, then be prepared to have life impose its terms on you. One must be able to see clearly the objectives desired and focus only on those objectives.

For every task, ask, "Is this helping to meet the objective?" If the answer is yes, then do it; if not, then do not. This is what focusing is all about. With constant focus on goals and objectives, the future will see each of them accomplished. A key element to success in the future will be the ability to articulate the quality difference between your agency and the competition's. To be able to control costs through a prevention-based strategy and to maintain the preferred work force will be competitive advantages of the future.

Tools

Visualization is a most powerful tool and the reason continuous quality improvement uses it extensively. People think in pictures; they respond to pictures; they understand pictures. Goals give drive, energy, direction, and focus. Goals assembled into a visual format provide an extremely valuable tool. The charts and graphs of continuous quality improvement will assist all staff members to keep the vision of improvement uppermost in their minds. Whether in quality improvement or daily life, there are five basic elements of success:

1. consistently outperform the competition
2. have a passion for excellence
3. express compassion for people
4. focus on objectives
5. plan for the future

If these strategies can be visualized and kept in focus, then success will be achieved.

Skills

Having the skills to do the job required will make excellence happen. Developing skills is synonymous with personal growth. Growing old is mandatory, growing up is optional, growing better is what everyone should accomplish. Success factors for an individual are slightly different from the five basic elements of success. Individuals need to be successful to accomplish the goals and objectives. It is up to management to create the environment within which individuals can motivate themselves for individual success. In order to do so, management should understand that individuals need:

- to have a vested interest
- to be rewarded for performance
- to be measured by specifics that are known to the individual

Skills in the new "world market" will provide a competitive advantage for both companies and individuals. Training and education are the cornerstones to greater consistency, which is the cornerstone for quality. Training typically deepens knowledge a person already has about a subject.[5] The methods of CQI are skills that can be acquired with an established base of knowledge.

> If the challenge were simply more choices and a faster flow, we could meet it with more organization and more speed—that is, with traditional time management and greater productivity. But we are also dealing with a rogue element: new choices, possibilities that have not been seen and dealt with before. Preprogrammed solutions, habits and previous personal experience may not work. Peak performers recognize that they are making not merely more choices, but new choices as well. The skills for handling "more and faster" do not always work with "new." . . . New requires learning, training, experimentation and integration.[6]

Statistical thinking and process control, the tools of quality, are the new rogue elements in health care. The skills necessary to harness these rogue elements can be acquired with education, training, and a desire to learn. H.G. Wells once said, "Statistical thinking will one day be as necessary for efficient citizenship as the ability to read and write."

Part of creating the environment for CQI is to provide employees with a general understanding of statistical thinking and methods. These are powerful tools in helping to identify action opportunities for continuing improvement, but the wisdom to use the education is also needed.

To transcend excellence will require more and more knowledge as the business environment becomes increasingly competitive. Only substantive knowledge can bridge the gap between what is and what can be.

THE ROLE OF EMPLOYEES

Every employee should feel that the corporate culture is one of continuously improving quality, and one that provides ever-improving value to customers. Every day, employees should ask themselves, What did I improve today? What did I learn today?

Employees are at their best when they are essential members of an organization that challenges them and accepts their ideas for improvement and growth, and allows them the opportunity to build individual successes as well as corporate successes.

Employees who perform a certain task know best how to improve that task, how to improve productivity, and how to be more efficient. All of these improvements must be encouraged by the agency and rewarded accordingly. When employees feel they are essential members of the team, their performance will bring about the quality–productivity connection!

NOTES

1. A.H. Maslow, A Theory of Human Motivation, *Psychological Review* (July, 1943).

2. D. McClelland, *The Achieving Society* (Princeton, N.J.: VanNostrand Reinhold & Co., 1961).

3. V.H. Vroom, *Work and Motivation* (New York: John Wiley & Sons, 1964).

4. L. Porter and E. Lawler's model of expectancy theory that expanded the original Vroom theory.

5. W.W. Scherkenbach, *The Deming Route to Quality and Productivity, Road Maps and Road Blocks* (Washington, D.C.: George Washington University, 1988).

6. C. Garfield, *Peak Performers* (New York: William Morrow & Company, Inc., 1986).

Chapter 7
Strategic Quality Planning

Strategic quality planning is an indicator of the degree to which agencies are willing and committed to implementing quality improvement. As previously stated, strategic quality planning should be integrated with business planning and focus on a long-term horizon while building in incremental steps, goals, and improvements for the short term.

The plan should be driven from aggressive benchmarks derived from studies of best in industry, best in class, and world-class. The plan must cover all services delivered by the agency and any products offered to the public. Products could be durable medical equipment, pharmacy products, etc. In developing the strategic quality plan, key targets or goals should be derived from customer requirements as identified from continuing research. Customer requirements include not only the needs of today but probable future needs.

Issues should be addressed that relate to integration of the plan throughout the organization. Integration will be assured based on how well each office, department, or individual employee assists in the achievement of the plan. The plan should also address suppliers, contractors, and other related groups upon whom the agency depends to supply products or services.

A method to ensure all aspects discussed should be covered within the framework of the strategic quality plan. The recommended method is *three-dimensional planning.*

THREE-DIMENSIONAL PLANNING

The integration of strategic quality and business planning will require a systematic method to assure the desired results. One such method is three-dimensional planning and consists of three elements: (1) approach, (2) deployment, and (3) results.

Approach

While all three planning elements are critical to the success of the strategic quality plan, *approach* will drive all other aspects and elements of the plan. The other two elements, deployment and results, must be linked to the approach. The approach refers to how the agency will achieve its quality and business objectives. The approach should be prevention-based. For example, a prevention-based approach to quality improvement would be to train appropriate staff in statistical process control and root cause analysis.

The approach should build in monitoring and evaluation cycles. For example, if the approach to customer satisfaction is to identify key quality characteristics, how often are these reviewed in relation to changing customer requirements? How are these requirements projected to change in the future? How are these determinations made?

The approach to continuous quality improvement (CQI) and total quality management (TQM) would be to utilize tools, techniques, and methods. This approach may be translated into the strategic quality plan as developing a "learning organization," building self-managed work teams, and empowering the work force to satisfy customers. The specific tactics and strategies for achieving these objectives are also covered in the approach.

In order to integrate the approach to continuous improvement throughout the organization, an organizational plan must be developed. While any number of organizational plans will work, for this discussion, we will refer back to Figure 1–5 in Chapter 1. This organizational plan looks at the agency cross functionally and touches every aspect of operations.

Deployment

The next key element to the strategic quality plan is how the agency will deploy or implement the plan throughout the organization. Deployment issues cover all transactions with customers and suppliers or contractors. Deployment begins with the approach and applies it to every service offered by the agency, including products that may be available to patients or others. For example, if the approach to improving customer relationships is to identify key quality characteristics, the tactic may be to implement relational quality strategies, including lateral service. The deployment would be through behavioral-based standards of performance measured and tracked by each operating unit or department. Employees would be trained in these strategies and evaluated on meeting the standards of performance. Rewards and recognition would be given according to performance.

Deploying quality initiatives throughout the organization includes all business functions. Often, agencies overlook the importance of office functions in the satisfaction of customers. Billing errors can cause as much dissatisfaction as any other mishandled customer contact. Deployment should, therefore, cover all functions and processes, even those—such as payroll—that may not interact directly with external customers.

Deployment strategies should also cover public interactions and responsibilities. For example, how does the agency handle indigent care? How responsibly does the agency react when insurance coverage reaches its limits and the patient is still in need of skilled care? Other issues involving public accountability, such as biohazardous waste disposal and proper discarding of chemotherapeutic agents, should be addressed.

Results

The last element of strategic quality planning is the result of the first two. The results are derived from the approach deployed. If results cannot be traced to the approach, there is no evidence to support either sustaining the outcome or the ability to replicate it. If the outcome can neither be sustained nor replicated, results are little more than an anomaly with no substantive foundation.

The desired results should be evidenced by goals in quality and performance levels that go beyond incremental improvement. While incremental improvement is a desired outcome, the home care industry must achieve "leapfrog" improvements to catch up with the quality levels necessary in today's competitive market. The rate of improvement should be sustained over time and seen in comparison to appropriate benchmarks.

Benchmarks have been addressed several times within this text. This concept shall be more fully explored within the context of the strategic quality plan.

BENCHMARKING

Benchmarking is a key route to breakthrough thinking. It opens windows to new ideas and ways of doing business. It establishes the opportunity for a paradigm shift, generally brought about through the "shock value" of seeing something work that you may have believed was impossible. Benchmarking highlights the gaps between what is and that which is possible. The improvement opportunities from benchmarking are enormous—which is why large consulting practices have grown up around this issue.

Benchmarking is an opportunity to learn. Years ago, benchmarking would have been called corporate espionage. In the more open and cooperative environment of total quality, benchmarking has become a way of life. In fact, one of the indicators of good business practice today is a company's willingness to share information with other companies. This is not to say that proprietary information is freely shared. What it does mean is that companies are more open about processes they have gone through to accomplish certain objectives. Generally, the process includes the company's approach, the deployment of the approach, and the results achieved.

For a benchmarking program to be successful (to feed the strategic quality plan), agency administrators should identify an area for improvement. This area should be a process or function where significant improvement is warranted. There are three levels of benchmarking as defined by Spendolini:[1]

Level 1. A broad area or subject of investigation. This level will give leadership a feel for the possibilities using the broad approach of total quality management (TQM), for example. Companies that have won the Malcolm Baldrige National Quality Award host leadership from other companies and present high-level overviews of their quality strategies. Level 1 benchmarking is recommended for the highest levels of leadership within the home care agency since it provides the opportunity to experience world-class quality.

Level 2. When leaders return from a level 1 benchmarking presentation, they will usually be excited enough about some aspects of it to initiate further study. Level 2 is the benchmarking of an activity or process, such as the customer service program, employee suggestion program, or the scheduling process of a widely disbursed mobile work force. This level of benchmarking would require an agency specialist in the subject matter under investigation.

Level 3. This level provides the greatest payback for the investment of time and money in benchmarking. As in level 2, agency specialists in the subject matter are required to perform this type of benchmarking. This level investigates specific tasks or functions that are generally defined with some measure or standard of performance. For example, if it cost the agency $3.26 to produce a UB–82, they may want to benchmark a company specializing in billing that has a production cost of 83 cents per claim form.

The identification of benchmark partners is another aspect to consider. How do you know which companies are the best in the industry, best in class, or world-class? Just because a company is considered world-class does not necessarily mean they are best in class in certain subject matters. For example, the Ritz Carlton is a world-class company as evidenced by their winning the Malcolm Baldrige National Quality Award. However, they are not best in class on the application of statistical process control in service industries. The best way to find out "who's who" to benchmark is to inquire at professional conferences or associations, review professional journals, and talk to people outside the home care and health care industry.

As stated previously, benchmarking can help the agency to see what is possible. It helps to establish the "leapfrog" goals necessary to significantly improve the operations. Benchmarking, therefore, drives the establishment of these stretch goals that should be built into the strategic quality plan. The approach to achieving these goals may also require benchmarking outside the home care industry.

If an agency chooses to use the organizational structure for strategic quality planning as identified in Chapter 1, Figure 1–5, then each of the strategies or overall approaches should be identified for each of the seven categories. For example, for customer service, the strategy may be the agency's long-term plan to offer an absolute service guarantee. The service guarantee would be considered the strategic initiative. How to accomplish this strategic initiative would be considered the tactical initiative. For example, to accomplish the strategy of a service guarantee, we may use the establishment of lateral service as the tactical initiative. We may also choose to further our tactical initiatives by adding a recovery strategy that supports adding value to ensure the absolute satisfaction of customers. (These issues were discussed in Chapter 4.) Figure 7–1 illustrates the concept of establishing strategies and tactics by organizational responsibility.

QUALITY ASSURANCE (QA) AND IMPROVEMENT PLANNING

While all the excitement over CQI and TQM leads health care providers to believe that the old QA is dead, nothing is further from the truth. Our business is health care and as such, we must never lose sight of the fact that our responsibility is to improve the outcomes of patient care. This issue was discussed earlier in this text. The strategic quality plan, while it must be integrated with business and improvement planning, must also include the more traditional components of planning for improvement in the outcomes of patient care.

Each agency must determine the scope of the strategic quality planning program by developing an overall plan to cover all activities and to designate the responsible parties for carrying out such activities. As a general rule, strategic quality planning involves stating a purpose for each activity and its review scope. Remember the overall objective of the plan should be to improve patient outcomes.

Strategic quality planning should consist of at least the following elements and focus on the resolution of identified or suspected problems that impact directly or indirectly on patients or on areas with potential for substantial improvements in patient care:

• purpose and objectives of program
• scope of program

STRATEGIC INITIATIVES

Leadership	Quality Planning	Information Analysis	Process Improvement	Human Resource	Customer Service	Results
CULTURE	DEVELOP-MENT OF PLAN	MEASURE-MENT SYSTEM	PROCESS OWNERS	EMPLOYEE CERTIFICATION PROGRAM	ABSOLUTE SERVICE GUARANTEE	25% MARKET SHARE
		QA SYSTEM	SUGGESTION PROGRAMS	REWARDS/ RECOGNITION		
			SUPPLIER CERTIFICATION PROGRAM			

TACTICAL INITIATIVES

EDUCATION	MBNQA	COST OF QUALITY PROGRAM	CYCLE TIME REDUCTION	CHARACTER TRAIT TECHNOLOGY	LATERAL SERVICE
POLICY	ISO 9000	KEY QUALITY CHARACTER-ISTICS	ERROR RATE REDUCTION		
COMPENSA-TION					

Figure 7–1 Critical Success Factors for Achievement of World-Class Status

- responsibility assignments and accountability
- implementation activities
    1. important aspects
    2. key indicators
    3. thresholds for evaluation
    4. data collection/sources
- monitoring and evaluation
- follow-up plans
- reporting mechanism/communication chain

The Joint Commission on Accreditation of Health Care Organizations (Joint Commission)[2] has changed its standards to incorporate the concepts of quality improvement. The standards changes will continue over several years. The Joint Commission's revised standards are based on the following principles:

1. The home care organization can improve patient care quality, e.g., increase the probability of desired patient outcomes by assessing and improving processes that most affect patient outcomes.
2. Some of the processes are carried out by clinicians, others are not.
3. Whether carried out by clinicians or others, all processes must be coordinated and integrated.
4. The opportunities to improve processes occur more frequently than do mistakes. Without abdicating its responsibility to address problems, the home care organization's principle goal should be to help everyone involved to improve processes.

The Joint Commission has recognized the weaknesses in the old approach to QA activities and is leading the way to encourage the profession to use models of continuous improvement. The overall goal of improving patient care outcomes is, however, intact.

Responsibility

The Joint Commission has changed the language in its standards from "delegation of responsibility" to language that identifies the organization's leaders as holding the responsibility for quality improvement. Leaders are defined as the leaders of the governing body, senior management, and other managers, as appropriate. However, while management is responsible for the overall program, specific components should be delegated to those who have daily operational authority. Department heads or other decision makers are preferred as accountable parties and would fit the language of leaders under the Joint Commission's definition.

Scope of Services

The scope of services should be focused but comprehensive so as not to overlook any potential for improvement. As previously discussed, the program should focus on improved outcomes of care. Additionally, a comprehensive approach could expand this clinical focus to improved outcomes for the downstream customer (i.e., the end user)—either internal or external.

Important Aspects of Care

The aspects of care most important to the health and safety of patients should be monitored and evaluated. These aspects would include the high risk, high volume, and problem-prone areas in each agency. The aspects of care are patient related. They can be considered the standards of care.

Indicators

Identifying the indicators to be monitored and evaluated is the key to the quality program, whether it is QA or CQI. In nonclinical settings, the indicators are referred to as key quality characteristics. By whatever name, the indicators identify the standards of practice and are caregiver related in clinical settings.

While there are no specific requirements for indicator development, it is suggested that agencies minimally address the following elements of an indicator to ensure an adequate understanding of what is being measured:

- a statement describing the indicator
- the aspect of care the indicator relates to
- the type of indicator
- the elements that make up the indicator
- the data source
- the frequency of monitoring

The Joint Commission, having done more work on indicator development than any other organization, has the following suggestions as to the issues to cover in the development of clinical indicators:

- indicator identification
- definition of terms
- type of indicator
  1. sentinel versus rate based
  2. process versus outcome
- rationale
  1. why useful
  2. supportive references
  3. components of patient care assessed
- description of indicator population
  1. patient subpopulations
  2. indicator logic
  3. indicator data format
- data element sources

- underlying factors
  1. patient factors
  2. nonpatient factors
- existing data bases[3]

Thresholds for Evaluation

Thresholds are the triggering mechanism for further evaluation to improve care. Thresholds can be stated in the positive or negative. For example, a threshold of 5 percent urinary tract infections on catheter patients could trigger further investigation as to the cause or, stated another way, 95 percent of patients with indwelling catheters should be infection free. The use of thresholds allows the agency to focus on only those events or processes that offer the opportunity for improved outcomes. The setting of thresholds, however, does not negate the agency's responsibility to perform surveillance to determine acceptable levels of a given issue. Thresholds are organization related and can be considered standards of performance. Exhibit 7–1 clearly illustrates the differences between the aspects, indicators, and thresholds.

Data Collection

Tools for the collection and organization of data related to the quality assurance and improvement program are not mandated by any party, which is probably the reason so few exist relative to home care. Proposed audit tools and statistical tools detailed within this book will assist the agency to fully document

---

Exhibit 7–1 Differences in Standards

ASPECTS	INDICATORS	THRESHOLDS
Standards of Care	Standards of Practice	Standards of Performance
(Patient related)	(Employee related)	(Organization related)

Source: Courtesy of Paula Swain, MSN, CPHQ.

efforts to improve care. This component of care planning deals with the data source; i.e., where can the needed data element be found? The data source should be clearly identified for any surveillance procedure.

Evaluation of Care

The process of auditing (surveillance) can only identify where problems or opportunities exist for improved outcomes. The heart of a CQI initiative is in the evaluation and analysis of the data collected and trended. Again, like all the other steps, this one need not be limited in scope to the clinical areas. The statistical tools detailed in Chapter 2 can be an enormous help in analyzing data to improve processes. It should be noted that any problems identified by the thresholds will generally require root cause corrective action in the process that produced the results rather than with an individual. This issue is at the very heart of CQI.

Actions

The specific action plan should be formulated to resolve the problem identified by the evaluation of the data. Again, the action must address root cause in the process in order to prevent recurrence and sustain an improvement.

Evaluation of the Actions

This step will ensure that the actions taken have had their desired result and will require the surveillance procedures to start over at the data collection step. Statistical methods are a must to validate the improved outcome and should be linked to the approach taken for improvement.

Communication

This component of the plan is often overlooked or underemphasized. Documentation is an important step in the communication process.

How many times have nurses been told, "If you didn't write it, you didn't do it"? The same holds true for the CQI effort. External review organizations, whether they have their basis in statutory authority or voluntary authority, require documentation of quality system actions and results. Careful consideration should be given to the confidential nature of these reports, to whom they will be sent, and the form or format of the communication.

All these issues will be worked out in the body of a strategic quality plan.

DEVELOPING THE PLAN

When developing the clinical portion of the plan, an agency should appoint a quality assurance and improvement committee. The committee should be composed of representatives covering the scope of services provided and any significant outside sources. For example, if the agency performs a large number of physical therapy visits, a therapist should be included on the committee. Likewise, if the agency has substantial referrals from a specific hospital, a representative from that facility should be invited to attend committee meetings. The committee should be made up of employees who have decision-making power and can orchestrate change.

The first task of the quality assurance and improvement committee should be to establish the clinical improvement plan and submit its contents for approval to the professional advisory board and the board of directors who will combine it with business planning. Each of the following components of the plan will become the quality assurance and clinical improvement program.

Purpose and Objectives of the Program

The purpose of a clinical quality assurance and improvement plan is to improve patient care outcomes through the identification and resolution of problems. It also serves to validate that the quality of care is consistent with agency standards and nationally recognized standards of care through the utilization of the nursing process. For agencies that will take a broader view, the purpose should be stated as improved outcomes for the downstream customer.

When trying to determine the purpose of the program, ask the question: What is the program intended to accomplish? The answer should provide insight to the purpose.

The objective of the quality assurance and improvement program should be stated in broad general terms focused on improved outcomes:

1. To establish a methodology that monitors and evaluates the clinical quality program and encompasses all functional areas impacting on the quality of patient care, resulting in improved outcomes of such care.
2. To identify strengths attesting to the quality of care and deficiencies in patient care delivery.

3. To document the needed improvement in processes and provide follow-up evaluation and consultation to ensure such improvements are implemented, consistently maintained, and improved.
4. To monitor the performance of caregivers juxtaposed to the standards of care for a stated diagnosis and incorporate such monitoring activities into the evaluations of staff (either probationary, annually, or for advancement purposes).
5. To monitor and continuously improve processes through the use of statistical methods.

Scope of the Program

Determining the program's scope is one of the most difficult development problems to face. The scope should be agreed on by all concerned parties, including the staff, the committee, the professional advisory board, and the board of directors.

The program scope will determine those areas to come under review. For a comprehensive program, the following recommendation is offered: The scope of the quality assurance and improvement program is to assess, evaluate, and improve customer outcomes through use of standardized criteria based on objective data sources.

If the agency chooses to limit the program's focus to patient outcomes, the types of activities should be defined as part of the scope:

- Appropriate professional practice shall be validated.
- Appropriate utilization of services shall be validated.
- Appropriate techniques of home care shall be validated.
- Appropriate clinical record documentation shall be validated.

Each of these statements concerns the process of validation. It is important to note that validation in and of itself is a process that encompasses the following activities: (1) monitoring and evaluation, (2) problem identification, (3) implementation and training, and (4) evaluation of results.

Responsibility Assignments and Accountability

As previously stated, the overall responsibility for quality rests with the board of directors. Generally speaking, this group of individuals does not have the technical expertise to manage a quality assurance and improvement program on a daily basis. Therefore, the board usually assigns the daily operational issues to a quality assurance professional. This assignment in no way abdicates the board's responsibility; it is simply expeditious.

For those agencies that will be involved with a full-scale continuous quality improvement program, the board usually appoints a steering committee of top-level managers who will oversee and provide direction for the CQI movement. For smaller agencies, the quality assurance and improvement committee is generally the arm of the board in quality matters.

Whichever route the board chooses to oversee the quality program, account-ability must be directed. The quality discipline has become very technical with the incorporation of CQI and should have a central coordinating figure who is knowledgeable and can be an agent of change. Likewise, the committee members should be experts in their own areas so that the group is far more knowledgeable than any one individual. This synergistic approach will allow for greater cooperation and coordination.

It is recommended that the heads of at least those departments whose functions are included in the scope of the program be members of the committee. This would include the six services identified on the organizational structure: QA, utilization review, infection control, risk management, staff development, and customer service (see Chapter 1, Figure 1–4).

If the agency has a marketing or research/development department, it should also be represented on the committee. Additionally, if the scope of the quality assurance and improvement program covers the indirect events affecting the downstream customer, these should also be represented.

Each person on the committee should be accountable for a specific component of the program. With this type of direct accountability, each member becomes the change agent for his or her department or function. It is important to note that as change agents, the committee members may want to adopt the Havelock and Havelock approach.[4]

1. People must participate in working out their own programs of change in order for both attitudinal and behavioral change to occur.
2. Attention is given to the individual's attitudes, values, norms, and external and internal relationships, emphasizing that these may require alteration or re-education.
3. Any outside influence for change must interact and collaborate with the individual in the definition and resolution of the needed change.
4. Unconscious resistance that impedes change must be brought into con-sciousness for examination.
5. The methods and concepts of the behavioral sciences are used in order to effectively deal with change.

The classic change theory articulated by Lewin should be understood before the committee attempts to motivate any type of change:

- "Unfreezing"—As the word implies, people must be motivated to unfreeze their attitudes and move in the direction of change.
- "Different behavior"—A new level of behavior must be reached through cognitive redefinition.
- "Refreezing"—Newly acquired behavior is integrated into personality. This requires reinforcement by immediate feedback and becomes over-learned skills discussed in Chapter 6.[5]

The committee's ultimate accountability is the extent to which each member can be successful as a change agent and create the environment within which the staff can motivate themselves to accept the positive changes.

Implementation Activities

The activities necessary to implement the program should be designed to address the following areas:

1. identification of relevant or potential problems in the care of patients
2. objective assessment of problems in processes producing undesirable results
3. implementation of designated mechanisms to eliminate identified problems within the process
4. use of monitoring activities designed to ensure achievement, maintenance, and improvement of desired results
5. documentation of the effectiveness of the overall program

Let us take a closer look at each of these functional areas.

Identification of Relevant or Potential Problems in the Care of Patients

Problems may be identified by various sources including—but not limited to—data sources, such as audit results, physicians, nursing and rehabilitative staff, senior and middle management, and any other employee or contractor. Each member of the agency's staff is responsible for ensuring that the highest quality of care is being delivered to the patient. When a staff member identifies a potential problem, it should be discussed with the immediate supervisor, who should set into motion one or more of the following processes:

- specific process-oriented studies, such as a diagnosis-related audit
- utilization review

- clinical record review
- review of adherence to corporate policy or procedural standards
- incident reports where indicated

Data collected should be measured in relation to the established standard on the specific tool utilized, providing a screening criterion in each area of service or function. The screening criterion will identify variations in care that can be trended to establish patterns of practice.

For example, the risk manager identified that many patient falls are a result of ambulating patients without using a safety belt. The quality assurance and improvement committee decided to do an on-site check of each employee to determine how many were noncompliant with the policy of ambulating unsteady patients with safety belts. It was determined that only 76 percent of the employees were using safety belts consistently. The agency's standard for an acceptable threshold was 98 percent compliance.

Clearly, the problem was in the staff's inconsistent compliance with appropriate technique as designated by the agency's procedure. The agency prioritized this issue and held an inservice plus subsequent individual follow-up visits with nurses and paraprofessionals. The same issue was retested after 90 days with the results showing 100 percent compliance; i.e., client care had an improved outcome as a direct result of the quality assurance and improvement program. Additionally, there were fewer incident reports on patients falling, resulting in an improved risk factor for liability purposes.

It is of vital importance that staff members see the reporting mechanism not as punitive, but as a positive response to patient advocacy. The attitude of management in responding to problems identified by staff will play a key role in the success of the program. Managers must understand that the purpose of a quality assurance and improvement program is not to cast blame, but to resolve problems in order to improve patient care. Managers and supervisors should welcome the opportunity to improve care, which can only happen if staff members become willing participants in problem identification and resolution.

Objective Assessment of the Problems in Processes Producing Undesirable Results

The quality assurance and improvement committee approves the audit tools used to determine the screening criteria for problem identification to assure an objective assessment. The criteria will be stated in measurable terms, utilizing a threshold percentage of acceptability for each category. The audit tools are based on nationally recognized standards of care, federal and state regulations, or corporate policy and procedure. The committee will use the screening criteria on patients who fall within the scope of the particular audit or on a statistically valid random number of cases for generalized audits during the surveillance process. A statistically valid sample for a generalized audit could be 10 percent, for example, selected at random from all patient records. The test data are analyzed by the committee and compared with the threshold percentages. Problems are identified, trended where necessary, and prioritized according to their impact on patient care. Appropriate training and follow-up is initiated once the root cause has been determined. Specific examples of audits will be found in subsequent chapters.

Implementation of Designated Mechanisms To Eliminate Identified Problems within the Process

Recommendations for corrective actions will be made by the individuals or committee that assessed the problem. This action takes place with appropriate department heads in concurrence with members of the senior management staff and the board of directors.

Recommendations must be objective and factual with no trace of bias and must be multidisciplinary when appropriate. All recommendations must be agreed on by the parties who will ultimately be responsible for implementation and must address the root of the cause. To impose a recommendation on a staff member who does not agree will only result in a half-hearted effort. The desired outcome will not be achieved on a permanent basis.

Recommendations can be made in the spirit of compromise so long as the desired outcomes are achieved.

Use of Monitoring Activities Designed To Ensure Achievement, Maintenance, and Improvement of Desired Results

Quality improvement activities of the agency should be monitored as indicated by the quality assurance and improvement committee and agreed upon by the administration and the board of directors. Periodic re-audits will be necessary for evaluating the effectiveness of previous recommendations for improved patient and client outcomes.

Re-audit results that are the same or similar to the original audit indicates a problem in the quality improvement process, not just in the rendering of patient care. All too often the program can break down at this point.

When re-audit results are similar, the quality assurance and improvement plan or process of surveillance must be reevaluated. Again, the objective is to improve patient care. If the quality improvement program is not having this effect, then something is wrong. Generally, the problem will be in the process or the failure to identify the actual root cause.

For example, a home health aide service audit was conducted to determine aide compliance with assignment of tasks. The first audit revealed a 36 percent compliance factor with an 80 percent acceptable threshold. Audit results identified that nurses were assigning every task on the preprinted form without regard for individualization. The aides, therefore, did not pay attention to the assignments by nurses; they did what the patients needed or wanted. This behavior was a process problem and was clearly not appropriate, not to mention its noncompliance with federal Conditions of Participation.

The recommendations called for an inservice with the aides to teach the importance of conformance to the assigned tasks and an inservice with the nurses to teach the necessity of individualization of aide assignments, as well as periodic updates of those assignments. Another recommendation was to establish a new corporate policy to require an updated aide assignment at least every 60 days.

After both inservices and after the new policy went into effect, another aide service audit was conducted by the caregivers. The results were compiled by the quality assurance and improvement committee, which was astounded by results similar to the first audit. Comments from the committee ranged from "The aides don't care," to "It's not important to them."

The classic, nonproductive blame mechanism took over. When this is allowed to continue, the result is a no-win situation. The quality assurance and improvement committee should not concern itself with blaming others for poor results. All employees of the agency are in the same boat and must learn to row together.

An objective retrospect of the second aide audit showed the committee that during and after the inservices, more attention was focused on the new policy than on the real issue of appropriate assignments and adherence to same. In fact, the managers revealed that they were relentless in their pursuit of updated assignments; however, review of the contents was cursory. The aides were told to make sure an updated assignment was in every home, which they did. However, the aides still did not make an effort to follow the assignment. Everyone lost focus of the primary problem, and the results of the second audit reflected that dismal state. The committee was forced to go back and start over, focusing on the primary problem with appropriate subsequent follow-up by line management.

The lesson to be learned from this account is that when audit results are similar, a process problem exists that will prevent achievement of the desired audit results until the real problem is found and corrected.

Documentation of the Effectiveness of the Overall Program

The reporting mechanism for quality improvement activities shall be in compliance with directives of the administration and board of directors. All quality assurance and improvement plans, audits, summaries, and results must be maintained in the agency's files.

Information obtained through the ongoing review and evaluation of care and information about the impact of actions taken to resolve problems should be documented and integrated with the agency's overall quality assurance and improvement program. These records should become a part of the agency's annual evaluation.

The effectiveness of the quality assurance and improvement program is measured by improved audit results and improved performance evaluations. The community at large judges quality on the basis of reputation and performance. As the agency improves, patients become more satisfied. Patient satisfaction leads to physician awareness, which can lead to additional referrals.

Some routine data to collect and monitor for quality assurance purposes as well as the agency's annual evaluation are:

- admissions by diagnosis
- admissions by referral source and by location
- discharges by reason
- utilization by service category
- total visits per patient, per length of stay, by discipline
- staff productivity

Each of these statistical categories can give the quality assurance and improvement committee clues regarding trends. For example, the agency's norm is that fractured hip patients receive physical therapy for an average of 45 days, with 17 skilled visits. By watching these statistics, the committee can quickly determine when an outlier occurs that could be an indication of a possible problem. In this case, if a therapist was consistently discharging fractured hip patients after only three visits in seven days, you can be sure the patient was not receiving optimum care, nor were the outcomes of care achieved. The problem, however, can be identified and rectified very rapidly by timely review of the statistical reports.

In order for this system to work effectively, the agency should establish the norms by reviewing data for a specified period of time in limited categories, such as for high volume cases.

Implementation activities constitute the most detailed of all components in a quality assurance and improvement plan. These activities have the greatest impact on direct patient care. For this reason, the 80/20 rule that is discussed in Chapter 2 should be recognized.

The issues of aspects, indicators, thresholds, and data collection have been discussed. The determination of each of these issues will require consensus and staff buy-in. The best way to get acceptance is to allow a great deal of participation.

Monitoring and Evaluation

Most home care agencies are currently performing some type of QA function. Many of these providers, however, have not pulled these activities together into a comprehensive quality improvement program.

For example, almost every agency has some type of review of clinical notes, plans of treatment, or medical records on an ongoing basis. These activities can be pulled together into a concurrent medical record review process.

Further examples of monitoring and evaluation activities include the following:

- Patient care conferences between managers and staff rendering care can be held on a periodic basis for every patient.
- Every patient and/or family can be given the right to initiate the procedure for a grievance.
- A utilization review nurse can review services retrospectively rendered every 30 days on every patient prior to billing.
- Random phone calls can be made to patients to assess patient and family satisfaction with the services rendered, or to address concerns.
- Comprehensive clinical record reviews can be performed every 60 days and at discharge.
- Staff can attend monthly inservice programs to keep abreast of the latest developments in health care.
- Medical advisory meetings can be held quarterly with the medical director and all managers to discuss new policies and procedures for patient care.
- The utilization review committee can meet quarterly with the medical director to review a random sample of active and discharged patient records in order to determine the appropriateness of care.
- The quality assurance and improvement committee can meet quarterly to review audit results, to address specific problems, and to implement a process for improvement in the deficient areas.
- QA surveillance can be performed by diagnosis or problems on a periodic basis.
- The administrator can perform an in-depth audit of the branch operation to determine whether staff are complying with agency standards.
- The administrator or designee can conduct an annual survey of all hospital social services/discharge planning departments to ascertain the perception of adequacy, appropriateness, and quality of care rendered by the agency.
- Customer service questionnaires should be administered at periodic intervals.

From the preceding list, it is easy to see that monitoring the agency's performance for quality is a constant and ongoing process. The quality assurance and improvement plan, under each audit activity, should define the mechanism for evaluating any specific component.

Committee members are encouraged to use a summary form for documenting their activities and those of their staff. A sample form can be found in Exhibit 7–2.

Follow-Up Plans

The best quality assurance and improvement plans are little more than exercises in futility without appropriate follow-up. The follow-up plans are methods used to ensure that the interventions deployed during the implementation phase achieved the desired results and that those results were sustained over time.

The ability to sustain improvements over time is the ultimate indicator of an agency's success in continuous improvement. It cannot be emphasized enough that, in order to sustain improvements, the problem must be taken down to the root cause and the correction must be systematic or process oriented.

Follow-up plans should use the same surveillance tools, data sources, and methods as the previous study. By replicating the original study, the only differential should be the results from interventions. This allows more objectivity to evaluate the interventions chosen to correct the problems identified from the original study. Any change from the methods used in the original study will add an element of variation to the follow-up that will be difficult to isolate.

Reporting Mechanism/Communication Chain

At least a summary of all activities in the quality field should be reported to the board of directors. Additionally, reports should be circulated to those with a "need to know." Any written reports should take care to protect the confidential nature of the quality disclosures and should be limited in circulation. It is also a good idea to label such reports confidential and file accordingly. Trend reports, however, should have wide circulation within the agency.

The type of reports to the board will determine the perception of effectiveness and the degree of importance placed on the quality assurance and improvement program. It is recommended that reports be in graphic form to convey an abundance of information at a glance. The statistical tools will be very helpful in this regard.

Exhibit 7–2 QA Committee Activities Summary Report

Months of Audit				Date	
Activity				Signature	
Date of Audit	Type of Audit	Results	Recommendations		Follow-Up Action

Source: Courtesy of Vickie Trevarthan, RN, Stone Mountain, Georgia.

Tracking systems will be useful to the director of the quality assurance and improvement program to coordinate and follow up on unresolved issues. A simple tracking system may contain the following information:

- the identified problem
- when and how the problem was identified
- what actions will be taken
- who is responsible for the action
- when the problem will be re-evaluated
- comments regarding the effectiveness of actions

All reports should be based on data from objective, quantifiable studies of quality. Data represent the difference between fact and opinion and should be used accordingly. The transmission of these data, however, can cause a problem with understanding unless the committee recognizes that barriers exist to the communication process.

Environmental Barriers

Environmental barriers can include the obvious, such as multiple locations and long distances, but also can include some issues that are not readily apparent, such as:

- noise (interference)
- competition for attention
- time restraints
- managerial philosophy of the organization
- multiplicity of hierarchical levels
- power–status relationships
- unfamiliar terminology
- complexity of the message[6]

Personal Barriers

Communication can also be compromised by the individual's perceptions of the issues involved. Information is power. People are either threatened by it or empowered by it. At least ten personal barriers to effective communications have been identified:

- frame of reference
- beliefs (paradigms)

- selective perception
- jealousy
- fear
- evaluation of the source
- desire to maintain status quo
- semantics
- symbols
- empathy[7]

For communication to be effective, each of these barriers will have to be overcome or at least minimized to some extent.

Figure 7–2 illustrates the flow of the quality assurance and improvement plan from appointment of a committee to the resolution of problems.

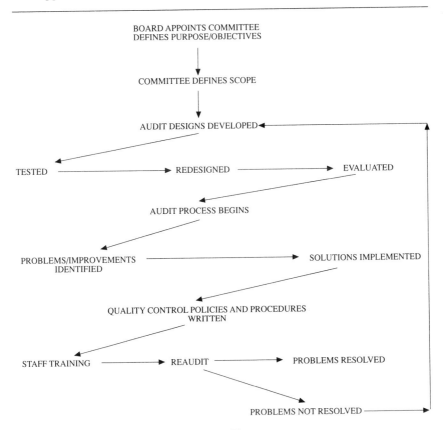

Figure 7–2 Quality Assurance and Improvement Plan

EVALUATION OF THE QUALITY ASSURANCE AND IMPROVEMENT PLAN

Agencies should evaluate the quality assurance and improvement program at least annually and revise it as indicated. This evaluation should include a review of the objectives, scope, organization, and effectiveness of the program.

Additionally, the National Association for Healthcare Quality, in its *Guide to Healthcare Quality Management,*[8] suggests that the following five components be included in the annual evaluation of the plan:

1. comprehensiveness
2. pertinence
3. validity
4. effectiveness
5. efficiency

Comprehensiveness

Evaluation of the plan should begin with questions such as: Is the plan comprehensive enough? Does it cover all services offered by the agency? Does it work cooperatively with all departments? Comprehensiveness should also include an inventory of statutory and regulatory requirements as well as other requirements from the specifiers using the Deming model.

Pertinence

What is important? Are the important issues being addressed? Has every service identified at least one outcome indicator that is monitored on an ongoing basis? Is the board of directors responsive to issues raised by the quality assurance and improvement committee? Are the plan data rich but knowledge poor? Have customers' most important aspects/indicators been considered?

Validity

The integrity of the program rests on the accuracy of identified problems and the resultant solutions. Some questions that should be asked are: What data sources are being used, and how reliable are those sources? What level of acceptance exists among the staff for the outcome criteria? Does the program have a reliable data collection and validation process? Are the data objective, quantifiable, and devoid of judgments? Is there any bias in the sample? Have the samples been chosen using statistically valid methods?

Effectiveness

The key to any evaluation of the quality assurance and improvement program is the response to the questions: Have we impacted positively on the outcome of patient care? Have we maintained or improved practice patterns? What important patient care problems have been resolved? Are there any outstanding issues not resolved?

Efficiency

Has the program optimally coordinated all efforts and data to the fullest extent to avoid duplication of efforts? Are meetings productive? Are the reports generated relaying useful information? Are initial results cost-effective? Has the program been cost-effective? What was the cost?

This efficiency component is the least understood aspect of the quality assurance and improvement plan. Very little work has been done in the area of quality costing. Concepts of "quality costs" were explained earlier. Yet, little is understood about the actual "cost of quality," because so little work has been done in this area.

The four categories of quality costs discussed earlier can be summarized into two groups.

1. costs of quality—the cost of preventative maintenance including surveillance and analytical studies
2. costs of lack of quality—the cost of system failure, rework, duplication, and surveillance for all occurrences[9]

As the industry matures in the concepts of continuous quality improvement, there will be additional specificity regarding this subject.

Once the plan is committed to paper, the committee should begin the process of quality improvement by developing the controls and teaching the staff the process of self-evaluation using those controlling standards. As a prerequisite for success, the plan must have a valid nucleus of information, a commitment from the staff, willing participation, a methodology based on uniform concepts, and well-developed outcome criteria.

NOTES

1. M.J. Spendolini, *The Benchmarking Book* (New York: American Management Association, 1992).

2. Joint Commission on Accreditation of Healthcare Organizations, *Manual for Home Care* (Oak Brook, Ill.: JCAHO, 1993).

3. K. Lewin, JCAHO Elements of Clinical Indicator Form (Oak Brook, Ill.: JCAHO, 1993).

4. R.G. Havelock and M.C. Havelock, *Training for Change Agenda* (Ann Arbor, Mich.: Institution for Social Research, 1973).

5. Attributed to Paula Swain, MSN, CPHQ at National Association of Professionals in Healthcare Quality Study Session, Atlanta, September, 1991.

6. National Association for Healthcare Quality, *Guide to Healthcare Quality Management* (Deerfield, Ill.: National Association of Professionals in Healthcare Quality, 1991).

7. J.S. Rakick, et al., *Managing Health Services Organizations* (Philadelphia: W.B. Saunders & Co., 1985).

8. National Association for Healthcare Quality, *Guide to Healthcare Quality Management,* 1991, p. 2:15.

9. W.E. Deming, *Out of Crisis* (Cambridge, Mass.: Massachusetts Institute of Technology, 1982).

Chapter 8

Auditing Types

Setting priorities and focusing on patient outcomes are important prior to determining the types of audits that an agency should be performing and the scope of the surveillance process. Each of these issues should be dealt with in the written quality assurance and improvement plan. Auditing is the method by which the patient care process can be monitored and subsequently improved.

AUDIT CATEGORIES

For the home care industry, there are two categories of auditing to be considered: (1) process audits and (2) outcome audits.

Process Audits

Process audits are methods of validation of events and procedures. It is a systematic method by which actions or behaviors can be judged objectively. It is the method by which a process can be monitored for improvement purposes. Process audits are almost always observed by a reviewer. These audits are the most difficult and time consuming, yet process audits exhibit the greatest results. An example of a process audit is the observation by the infection control nurse of another nurse performing a sterile dressing change. The reviewer in this case is personally validating that the nurse is changing the dressing in accordance with the written procedure and is technically competent.

A process audit therefore validates two components:

1. The nurse knows the written procedure (i.e., quality control).
2. The nurse performs the procedure with technical competence (i.e., concurrent quality assurance process of observing standards of practice).

Process audits become an excellent tool for staff development purposes and should be used when an employee is up for promotion, for evaluation, or when competence in a new technical procedure needs to be validated.

A process audit is also a valuable tool when validating the quality of the service delivery component of the entire agency.

Outcome Audits

Outcome audits are most closely associated with diagnosis-related auditing or other quality assurance audits in which expected outcomes denote specific interventions. Outcomes are the most significant result of quality assurance. This category of auditing is essential to validate quality based on nationally recognized standards of care. For example, an uncontrolled diabetic would require an outcome of stability with the interventions of teaching, diet control, and perhaps insulin or other medication.

An assumption is made that if the desired outcome is not achieved, there was a problem with the intervention. A quality assurance professional would look at the nursing care plan for any possible omissions in interventions that prevented the desired outcome from being achieved.

This category of auditing has the greatest impact on direct patient care and should be included in the quality assurance and improvement plan for the agency. However, for improvement to occur, the process that allowed a deficiency would require study.

AUDIT TIMING ELEMENTS

Before we discuss the specific types of audits, it should also be mentioned that the time span of audits will impact on the result an agency wishes to achieve. In this regard, there are three timing elements to consider:

1. retrospective
2. concurrent
3. prospective

Retrospective Audits

Retrospective audits are those audits performed after the fact. An example of an audit with this timing element would be a clinical record review for quality assurance purposes. Obviously, an audit of clinical records is completed after care is rendered and documentation is written. Another example of a retrospective audit is a discharged patient audit. Some retrospective audits, such as utilization review, while accomplished after the fact, can also impact on prospective outcomes.

Concurrent Audits

Concurrent audits take place during the course of treatment. They directly impact current care being rendered and could impact on future care to be rendered. These audits are considered the most effective. Field auditing is a good example of the concurrent audit process. Another useful concurrent audit is review of plans of treatment at the start of care, at the time of verbal orders, or at case conferences. Should a problem or an opportunity for improvement be noted, corrections or additions can be made that will improve client outcomes while the individual is still under care.

Prospective Audits

Prospective auditing is an underutilized opportunity. Prospective auditing in its finest form is a system of case management for optimal patient care. In this scenario, the case manager or reviewer projects into the immediate future the overall needs of the patient. For example, a cerebrovascular accident (CVA) patient is admitted to the agency for nursing, physical and speech therapy, and home health aides. During review, the case manager notes that the speech therapist has indicated the patient has difficulty handling the cue cards. The nurse recognizes this as a potential need for fine motor function therapy. After discussions with the physical therapist, a decision is made to ask the physician for an order for occupational therapy. Review for service utilization should also look at continuing and future services as well as coverage of past services.

Categories and timing elements can be confusing. Table 8–1 attempts to clarify these issues.

Now that categories and timing have been discussed, the specific types of audits can be reviewed.

QUALITY ASSURANCE AUDITS

Quality assurance is an audit process by which professional practice is validated utilizing nationally recognized standards of care by diagnosis or

Table 8–1 Audit Components

	Process Audits	Process/ Outcome Audits	Outcome Audits
Type	Field Review Audit	Administrative Review Audits	Quality Assurance Audits Utilization Review Audits
Timing	Concurrent	Retrospective	Retrospective (should project current and future care)

disease state. One of the most commonly used quality assurance mechanisms is nursing care related to the diagnosis, or the diagnosis-related audit. This type of audit is retrospective but can influence prospective outcomes. Since these audits are based on outcomes, the reviewer should identify opportunities for improvement when standard outcomes are not achieved.

The agency should look at which diagnoses should be audited. As a general rule, no more than ten diagnoses should be audited over an extended period of time. These diagnoses should include the top admitting diagnoses as well as the diagnoses rarely admitted. The reasoning behind this general rule is to audit high volume and low volume, which generally increases the risk. The high-volume diagnoses will cover the majority of clients within the agency, while the low volume diagnoses will cover the high risk clients. It is generally felt that if an agency does not do something often, there is a greater potential for error or increased risk.

In choosing the diagnoses to audit, the agency should review the admission patterns over at least a 12-month period. Generally, home care admissions by diagnoses do not fluctuate greatly. An influencing factor in the admission diagnoses fluctuation could be the addition of a new referral source. For example, if the agency has just signed a contract to provide home care for an orthopedic hospital, the number of admissions with orthopedic diagnoses will significantly increase.

For purposes of discussion, the following diagnoses will be used:

1. cerebrovascular accident (CVA)
2. congestive heart failure (CHF)
3. hypertension (HTN)
4. cancer (CA) (specific or general)
5. diabetes
6. chronic obstructive pulmonary disease (COPD)
7. decubitus ulcers

8. failure to thrive
9. Crohn's disease
10. acquired immune deficiency syndrome (AIDS)

It is important to remember that while ten diagnoses appear insignificant in relation to the hundreds of different diagnoses home care agencies treat annually, time will prohibit an agency from auditing all ten in any given year. Doing the actual audit is not the time-consuming part of the process. The largest portion of time will be spent in the training, follow-up, and re-audit.

It is suggested that the field nurses themselves perform the actual audit as a group with supervision from the quality assurance and improvement committee. This could be accomplished easily during a regularly scheduled inservice. The audit itself takes approximately 15 minutes. Nurses should trade off so as not to audit their own patient records. The compilation and interpretation of results should be the committee's responsibility, as should developing any follow-up activities necessary.

The purpose of allowing field nurses to perform the audit is threefold:

1. Through the process of auditing, nurses will learn (relearn) the standards by which they are being judged.
2. The nurses will have a better understanding of documentation requirements.
3. A large number of patient records can be audited in a very short period of time.

To begin the surveillance program, it is suggested that a diagnosis-related audit should be performed at least twice per year, with the ultimate goal of performance on a quarterly basis.

However, a second audit should not be undertaken until the entire cycle of the first audit has been completed—up to and including meeting the acceptable thresholds established by the agency for compliance. On the first audit, it may take the agency several months and many re-audits to accomplish the minimum compliance percentages.

It is also suggested that the field nurses complete diagnosis audits on clients who were admitted with the specific diagnosis under investigation. For example, if CVA is the first diagnosis audit performed by the agency, then only review those charts where CVA is the primary diagnosis. Do not review charts with CVA as a secondary or contributing diagnosis.

In order to validate the results of the audit by the field nurses, the quality assurance and improvement committee should re-audit a random sample of charts and compare the results to those of the field nurses. This process will ensure that the nurses were properly instructed in the completion of the audit tool and will substantiate that audit results are accurate.

The quality assurance and improvement committee should compile and interpret the results of the audit using the tools of statistical process control and report its findings to the professional advisory board (PAB) and the board of directors. Results should also be relayed to the nursing staff who participated in the audit. If the audit results are less than the established acceptable threshold, the committee will set into motion the process of evaluation of the problems, root cause analysis, process changes, subsequent training, and appropriate follow-up.

Specific examples of diagnosis-related audits are found in subsequent chapters.

UTILIZATION REVIEW AUDITS

The utilization review (UR) audit is a process by which appropriate utilization of services is validated in accordance with guidelines established by the payer source, including the efficient use of resources. These audits are the most common in home care since the majority of intermittent visits made are payable under the provisions of the Medicare (Title XVIII) or Medicaid (Title XIX) programs. Medicare mandates the UR function.

The Joint Commission requires that agency leadership take adequate steps to ensure the quality and appropriateness of services. Specific services to be provided to patients and actions to be taken to meet patient's needs are noted and periodically reviewed. These are utilization review functions.

Professional standards review organizations (PSROs) were charged with the responsibility to determine whether medical care provided in hospitals was necessary and had been provided in a cost-efficient manner. Not until the advent of a prospective diagnosis-related group (DRG) payment system did hospitals begin to place emphasis on the UR process. The PSROs were ultimately replaced with the current professional review organizations (PROs), which have review authority over home care. The PROs have more authority than did their predecessors. They have the power of sanction if the agency fails to comply with established guidelines. For these reasons, UR has become increasingly important.

UR audits can be either retrospective, concurrent, or prospective and are outcome based. However, when reviewing retrospectively, or after the client is discharged, the UR process loses some of its effectiveness. It is recommended, therefore, that UR audits be completed after documentation is completed but as early as possible in order to concurrently and prospectively project appropriate levels of care. In other words, UR audits are retrospective but should always project current and future levels of care in accordance with payer guidelines.

Because each entitlement program and third-party payer source has different rules and regulations, it is recommended that an audit tool be developed for each.

These audits should be payer-specific and deal with issues such as qualifying criteria, medical necessity, and frequency and duration of services juxtaposed to the patient's condition.

Unlike the diagnosis-related audit, the UR audit process allows a reviewer to use the "judgment call." Generally speaking, a judgment call during an audit process is not good practice since different people have different opinions based on experience and knowledge. For an audit to have the optimum result, all subjectivity should be removed, allowing only for objective fact-based findings. Put another way, an objective or fact-based audit will have the exact same result regardless of who conducts the audit. Since the diagnosis-related audits are fact based, any nurse conducting the audit should come to the same conclusion.

This is not always the case in UR audits. For example, Medicare covers skilled intermittent care for a homebound patient. One fiscal intermediary may interpret the need for fasting blood sugars (FBS) to be drawn at a 60-day frequency while another intermediary may only allow an FBS at a 90-day frequency.

The experience of the UR reviewer and his or her knowledge of the intermediary or other payer will impact significantly on the effectiveness of the UR process. Although use of judgment calls may not be the best method for an audit, it is, however, necessary for utilization review.

The judgment call questions should have parameters within which the judgment can be made. For example, the question may be asked: Are skilled services evident in the record? Upon review of the clinical record, the reviewer finds that the nurse is monitoring vital signs on a hypertensive client under Medicare and that the blood pressure fluctuates between 160/100 and 190/110. Are skilled services evident? Before the question can be answered, the parameters must be established within which to make the decision:

- What was the extent of physician intervention?
- What interventions has the nurse implemented?
- How long has the blood pressure been within this range?
- How long has the agency been serving this client?
- Is the client symptomatic, newly on medication, or had a recent change in medications?

Once these questions have been answered, the reviewer can make a judgment. Again, judgment calls can be made by the reviewer but only after clear parameters or criteria have been established to provide a basis for an objective opinion.

The UR audit process should be completed on every patient at the start of care, when significant changes occur, and at the time of recertification. Because UR audits are subject to judgments, it is strongly recommended that the same person perform UR audits on a consistent basis.

FIELD REVIEW AUDITS

Unlike the other types of audits previously discussed, field reviews are process audits and are concurrent in nature.

The most common type of field review is the infection control audit. It is a process audit; the reviewer will observe as the nurse, therapist, or paraprofessional renders care. Issues such as handwashing technique and bag technique are validated, as well as technical procedure used with infectious clients or those requiring invasive procedures.

Additionally, the field review has become a tremendous asset to managers who must evaluate nurses and other field staff for performance or promotion. A portion of this audit should include a client questionnaire in order to make an objective determination regarding the teaching and communication skills of the nurse.

Since infection control, technical procedure, and patient interview audits are all performed in the home setting, it is recommended that the audits be combined for logistical and resource conservation purposes. The field review audit should be completed at least annually on all personnel and at such other times as necessary. The line manager can conduct this audit after appropriate training.

ADMINISTRATIVE REVIEW AUDITS

The administrative review is an audit process by which the clinical record is validated in accordance with established policies and procedures of the agency. These audits could be retrospective, concurrent, or prospective. They are both outcome and process oriented depending on the purpose of the specific audit.

A number of different audits can be performed under administrative review:

- branch or agency audit (retrospective/outcome)
- risk management audit (retrospective with prospective outcomes/process)
- client/employee/physician satisfaction surveys (retrospective/outcome)

The agency should decide the frequency of any audit under this type. The branch audit, for example, could be done on an annual basis while surveys to determine customer satisfaction could be done more frequently.

A risk management audit can be done in conjunction with a patient or employee incident report by the supervisor or risk manager who would report

Exhibit 8–1 Audit Types

	Quality Assurance	Utilization Review	Field Review	Administrative Review
Audit Method	Outcome	Outcome	Process	Process or Outcome
Audit Timing	Retrospective	Retrospective (should project current and future care)	Concurrent	Retrospective
Audit Specifics	1. Diagnosis-Related Audits (by diagnosis) 2. Service Audits	Utilization Review Audit	1. Infection Control 2. Staff Performance 3. Client Questionnaire	1. Branch Audits 2. Risk Management Audits 3. Client Satisfaction Questionnaire 4. Employee Questionnaire
Audit Frequency	Every 6 months	Every patient every 60 days	Every field employee annually and on promotion	1. Annually 2. As incidents occur 3. Upon discharge 4. Every 6 months
Audit Reviewer	Field Staff	Utilization Review (UR) Nurse	Manager or Supervisor	1. Administration 2. Quality Assurance and Improvement Committee

findings to the quality assurance and improvement committee. The specific incident is trended with other incidents to identify potentially unsafe patterns of practice or processes that should be improved. The branch audit is an overview of all policies and procedures of the agency. The audit purpose is to determine compliance by the individual manager or supervisor and to ensure procedures are in place as indicated by the scope of service. Since a significant part of determining quality relies on customer satisfaction, this type of audit tool (survey) is extremely useful in developing or changing agency policies and procedures. The employee satisfaction tools will help agencies develop benefit and compensation packages that will assist in recruiting and retaining good staff. Each of these issues is discussed in detail in this text.

Exhibit 8–1 identifies in visual form the different audit types and their component parts.

Chapter 9

Quality Assurance Audits

Quality assurance (QA) audits are the most exacting of all audit types and pay the biggest dividends in improved patient care. These audits are based on nationally recognized standards of care and outcome criteria, but can also be research-oriented if new techniques are being tested. An overview of the quality assurance audit follows:

- Who is the client population?
- What specifically will be audited?
- When will the audit cycle begin, and what period of time will it cover?
- Why are specific indicators selected?
- Where will data sources be located?

Each agency must answer these questions individually for every audit.

DEVELOPING THE AUDIT

Step 1: Scope of Care[1]

The first step delineates the therapeutic modalities used, procedures performed, or services provided and to whom, either by disease state, age group, or disability. For example:

Q: What types of patients are served?
(age, disability, diagnosis, case mix, etc.)
A: Medicare beneficiaries over age 70 admitted with primary diagnosis of cerebrovascular accident (CVA) with hemiparesis.
(answers who is the client population)

175

Q: What client services are delivered?
   (disciplines, frequencies, and specific therapies or modalities)
A: Nursing and physical and occupational therapy delivered at frequency of at least three times a week.
   (answers what services will be audited)
Q: At what point will the audit occur for outcome indicators to be evident?
A: At least 30 days after admission through 60 days of service.
   (answers when the audit begins and coverage period)
Q: What basic clinical activities are required?
A: Assessment, patient teaching, home exercise program, and follow-through.
   (answers why these specific indicators were selected)
Q: Where will the information be located?
A: Specific page references in clinical record where data are recorded.
   (answers where the data source is located)

Step 2: Significant Aspects of Care

Step 2 identifies the more important or significant aspects in therapeutic modalities that impact on the outcome of care. As previously mentioned, aspects of care relate to standards of care and are patient related. Clinical activities that involve a high volume of patients (for example, CVA), those that entail a high degree of risk to patients, or those that tend to produce problems for staff or patients should be deemed most important for purposes of monitoring and evaluation. The Joint Commission on Accreditation of Healthcare Organizations (Joint Comission) requires monitoring and evaluation of aspects of care that are most important to the health and safety of patients. Examples may include:

- medication administration
- specific standards of care

Each of these examples is a review element for which interventions are standardized and specific outcomes are expected.

Step 3: Clinical Indicators

An indicator is an objective, measurable variable relating to the structure, processes, or outcome of care. Indicators are standards of practice and relate to the caregiver. Indicators include structures, processes of care, and outcomes of care.

Structures are inputs into care such as resources, equipment, policy, procedures, and qualifications of staff over which the individual employee does not maintain direct control. These can also be the rules and regulations under which the care is rendered.

Processes of care are those functions carried out by nurses, therapists, etc., that are within the direct control of the staff person.

Outcomes of care include complications, adverse events, short-term results of specific procedures, and longer-term status of patients' health and functioning. The outcomes are those objectives sought after specific interventions.

In order to monitor the significant aspects of care in step 2, data must be collected for each of the above indicators. Therefore, these indicators should be measurable and well defined for ease and reliability of data collection. It should also be noted that data should always be collected from a consistent place or event. For example, define where the data are to be found, i.e., the first nurse's note, care plan, etc. This prevents reviewers from wasting time looking through the entire record when only one data element is required.

Indicators for the process of care are very often the standard of practice. Such indicators can include objective clinical criteria established by the agency based upon authoritative sources such as the clinical literature. In short, indicators are expectations for each aspect of care. The following are some helpful questions to ask when developing clinical indicators:[2]

- What is the indicator, and how is it operationalized?
- What data elements must be collected and from where?
- How are data elements defined and collected to ensure uniform application?
- What is the clinical rationale behind the indicator?
- What aspects of care does the indicator tap into?
- What factors could account for variation in indicator rates?

Step 4: Thresholds for Evaluation

The data collected for each indicator cannot alone lead to conclusions about the quality of care. The indicator can, however, direct attention to those areas in which a problem or other opportunity to improve care may be found. As data are collected over a series of cases or over time, there must be a preestablished level or point in the cumulative data that triggers a committee response for evaluation purposes. When reached, this threshold initiates the process of evaluation to determine whether an actual problem or opportunity to improve exists.

For example, a clinical indicator is established that a patient with systolic blood pressure on admission greater than 160 mm Hg or diastolic blood pressure greater than 95 mm Hg is to have a follow-up visit within 24 hours. The threshold for evaluation is set at 98 percent. That is, professional evaluation would be undertaken if in more than 2 percent of patients, a return visit within 24 hours was not done. The question, "What process needs improvement?" would have to be answered.

It is important to realize that thresholds apply to a specific indicator and should not be viewed as universally applicable to an audit as a whole, unless the audit is reviewing only one specific indicator. There are, of course, exceptions to every rule. Administrative audits generally apply thresholds to the entire audit. Thresholds for evaluation are the agency's standards of performance and are organizationally related.

The threshold for evaluation premise may begin with, "All occurrences warrant investigation..." but agencies do not have the time or financial resources to pursue all occurrences. Therefore, we must establish the types of events upon which to set thresholds:

1. Sentinel Event—a significant event that warrants further investigation at each occurrence. An unexplained patient death is an example.
2. Relative Rate Indicator—frequent events where trending is necessary to establish further assessment of a potential problem. These events would require a threshold for evaluation.

Exhibit 9–1 shows an example of going through each of the four steps.

This example deals with a specific nursing intervention. Medication administration in a stroke patient is a very important aspect of care. However, there are other aspects of care that can have a significant impact on the outcome of care as well. The next example, shown in Exhibit 9–2, will deal with a diagnosis more generalized and those important aspects of care that have the greatest impact on the outcome of care.

Scoring for all of the audits works essentially the same way. Total possible points to be allocated are in the far left column of Exhibit 9–2. The next column is for the actual score received to be written. Each part is scored separately and has a different threshold. If a question is not applicable, reduce the total possible points in that part by the total of not applicable points. Add up all actual points. Divide the actual points by the possible points to get the percentage. Compare this percentage to the threshold to determine whether the results are within acceptable limits.

Note that data sources are indicated on the audit tool and should be adhered to on all questions. If the response cannot be found at the data source location, the reviewer is instructed to indicate "no" on audit.

The point of the diabetes sample audit tool is to show that the five Ws have been addressed:

1. Who—insulin-dependent diabetic over 65 years
2. What—aspects of care that are most significant

Exhibit 9–1 Sample Audit Tool 1: Threshold for Evaluation

STEP 1: SCOPE OF CARE:

Medicare patient over age 70 admitted with cerebrovascular accident.

STEP 2: SIGNIFICANT ASPECTS OF CARE:

Medication Administration: Patient with medication as ordered to maximize health capabilities. (Standard of Care.)

STEP 3: INDICATORS:

Indicator: Medications are administered accurately according to procedures and physician orders.

1. Structure Indicator: The same nurse will teach medication administration.
2. Process Indicator: RN will teach signs and symptoms of medication toxicity, side effects, and emergency protocol.
3. Outcome Indicator: Patient will be able to return demonstration and knowledge of medication administration with 98% accuracy.

(Standard of Nursing Practice: The nurse will design intervention to promote, maintain, and restore health.)

Indicator: Medication errors.

1. Structure Indicator: Presence or absence of medication in the home.
2. Process Indicator:
   • Medication orders are written accurately.
   • Medications are administered per orders.
3. Outcome Indicator: The right patient receives:
   • the right medication
   • in the right dose
   • via the right route
   • at the right time

STEP 4: THRESHOLD FOR EVALUATION:

1. Structure Indicators: 85% compliance
2. Process Indicators: 98% compliance
3. Outcome Indicators: 98% compliance

---

3. When—review over a 60-day period
4. Why—most significant aspects impacting outcomes
5. Where—location of data sources identified

The same simple process can apply to any diagnosis-related or specific modality where a problem is perceived or an improvement in care is desired.

Exhibit 9–2 Sample Audit Tool 2: Diabetes Mellitus

SCOPE OF CARE:

- Diabetes mellitus (primary diagnosis)
- Patient newly insulin dependent over 65 years of age
- Admitted to agency within 60 days of onset and has been a patient for at least 30 days

SIGNIFICANT ASPECTS OF CARE:

1. Teaching process
2. Assessment process

CLINICAL INDICATORS:

1. Structure Indicators: Compliance with protocols outside the nurse's control
2. Process Indicators: Compliance with protocols within the nurse's control
3. Outcome Indicators: Result of indicators and patient compliance

THRESHOLDS (evaluation of clinical indicators):

1. Structure Indicators: 85% compliance
2. Process Indicators: 98% compliance
3. Outcome Indicators: 80% compliance

INSTRUCTIONS:

- Check yes when criterion has been met.
- Check no when criterion was not met.
- Check N/A when the criterion does not apply to the patient or when the patient's primary diagnosis changes as a result of an acute episode or document noncompliance. Surveyors are instructed to reduce the points allocated to N/A questions for threshold compliance.

Possible Points	Actual Points		Yes	No	N/A	Comments
		PART I: Structure Indicators (66 points)				
5		1. Does the record indicate that teaching was directed to the primary caregiver? Data Source: First 7 visit notes				
10		2. Are contents of home health aide (HHA) assignments individualized? Data Source: Last HHA assignment sheet				

Exhibit 9–2 continued

Possible Points	Actual Points		Yes	No	N/A	Comments
9	_____	3. Were safety measures identified as indicative of diagnosis? Data Source: Plan of treatment (POT)/ psychosocial factors				
8	_____	4. Is patient history reflective of primary diagnosis? Data Source: Nurse assessment (history)				
10	_____	5. Are the goals related to the primary diagnosis?				
4	_____	a. Are the stated goals measurable?				
4	_____	b. Are they stated with a time frame? Data Source: POT				
6	_____	6. Is equipment identified? Data Source: Psychosocial factors of RN assessment				
10	_____	7. Is care plan reflective of primary diagnosis?				

Total
Points: Thresholds:
66 _____   85% _____

Possible Points	Actual Points		Yes	No	N/A	Comments
		PART II: Process Indicators (237 points) 1. Does the record indicate patient/caregiver was taught:				
16	_____	a. Insulin preparation				
16	_____	b. Insulin administration				
11	_____	c. Rotation of sites				
16	_____	d. Blood sugar monitoring				
16	_____	e. Diet management				
15	_____	f. Signs/symptoms of hypoglycemia				
15	_____	g. Signs/symptoms of hyperglycemia				

continues

Exhibit 9–2 continued

Possible Points	Actual Points		Yes	No	N/A	Comments
15	_____	h. Emergency measures				
13	_____	i. Weight control				
12	_____	j. Skin care				
12	_____	k. Foot care				
12	_____	l. Mouth care				
9	_____	m. Activity to promote circulation				
8	_____	n. Signs/symptoms of local or systemic infections				
8	_____	o. Other complications Data Source: First 30 days of service nurses' notes except emergency measures, which should be on first visit note				
15	_____	2. Were identified safety measures taught? Data Source: Nurse's notes first 7 visits				
8	_____	3. Was equipment checked for safety? Data Source: Psychosocial factors				
20	_____	4. Was care plan updated with pertinent changes and with dates and initials?				

Total Points:		Thresholds:	
237	_____	98%	_____

Possible Points	Actual Points		Yes	No	N/A	Comments
		PART III: Outcome Indicators (247 points)				
40	_____	1. Does the record indicate that fasting blood sugar levels are maintained between 65–125 mg/dL unless physician orders specify different parameters? Data Source: Lab results after 14 days of service				

Exhibit 9–2 continued

Possible Points	*Actual Points*		Yes	No	N/A	Comments
		2. Does the record indicate that				
20	____	a. Patient or caregiver prepares insulin doses correctly?				
20	____	b. Patient or caregiver administers injection correctly?				
		3. Does the record indicate that:				
20	____	a. Patient verbalizes understanding of diet?				
19	____	b. Weight is stable +/– 2 lbs unless weight gain/loss is desired Data Source: 4th week of service nurses' notes				
18	____	4. a. Does the record indicate that skin is intact?				
17	____	b. If skin breakdown is evident, was treatment plan initiated? Data Source: Nurse's notes				
16	____	5. Record indicates mouth is clean and dental problems referred as necessary? Data Source: Nurse's notes				
15	____	6. Does the record indicate that patient or caregiver rotate sites correctly? Data Source: Nurse's notes				
14	____	7. Does the record indicate that foot care has been implemented as taught? Data Source: Nurse's notes				
		8. Does the record indicate that:				
12	____	a. Blood pressure is maintained between 90/60 and 160/90 mm Hg				
12	____	b. Pulse is 60–90 beats per minute and regular				
12	____	c. Respiratory rate is 12–24 breaths per minute at rest and unlabored				

continues

Exhibit 9–2 continued

Possible Points	Actual Points		Yes	No	N/A	Comments
12	____	d. Temperature is 96.4–99°F orally (unless physician orders are evident with specific parameters to the contrary) Data Source: Nurse's notes				
		Instructions to #8: If vital signs are outside of stated parameters, the auditor may still give points if the record indicates that the nurse noted the change, recorded an explanation, and intervened with notification to the physician.				
Total Points: 247	____	Thresholds: 80% ____				

Source: Courtesy of Vickie Trevarthan, RN, Stone Mountain, Georgia.

Part I of the audit for structure indicators is generic and can apply to any other diagnosis-related audit. Further examples of diagnosis-related audits are found at the end of this chapter.

COMPARING QA TO QUALITY IMPROVEMENT

Many QA professionals are probably worried over the prospect of having to "start all over again" with the concepts of continuous quality improvement (CQI). Some may even be worried about all those numbers required in data analysis and trending. The nurses who have steadfastly held the banner for quality all these years may feel threatened by the new (and probably nonclinical) quality professional. All of these fears and worries should be put aside, because there is room for all to be active participants in the new quality discipline.

This new quality discipline is changing from subjective to objective, from qualitative to quantitative, from opinions to data, from individualizing problems to process problems, from limited access to broad access, from clinical issues to all issues, and from patients to customers. All of these changes will improve patient care and all outcomes for every customer.

We are on the threshold of the development of a new medical discipline. Quality improvement has become the science of change and of knowing what needs to be changed and when. Quality professionals will know what questions to ask based on statistical evidence.

Exhibit 9–3 illustrates the differences between quality assurance and quality improvement. It is comforting to know that CQI will expand QA rather than starting over. Exhibit 9–4 was reprinted from the *Guide to Health Care Quality Management* and compares quality assurance and quality improvement using the Joint Commission's 10 step model.

Exhibit 9–3 Characteristics of Quality Assurance and Quality Improvement

QUALITY ASSURANCE	QUALITY IMPROVEMENT
Organized according to organizational structure	Organized according to processes (i.e., patient care)
Leadership rarely comes from top management and is delegated to a few	Leadership from the top and delegated to all
Conflicts over the definition of quality	Quality = customer satisfaction
Little guidance and, consequently, similarity in quantitative methods or display	Quantitative methods and displays based on accepted statistical principles
Detection orientation	Prevention orientation
Thresholds for evaluation (data points)	Control limits (data ranges)
Adversarial. Indicators which meet thresholds for evaluation too easily lead to questions like: Who's responsible and what should be done to them?	Collegial. Variation causes the questions: Why did it happen (chance vs. assignable cause) and how can we work together to improve it?
Primarily focused on problem resolution	Primarily focused on continuous improvement
Rarely integrated determination of quality with efficiency (cost)	Quality cost measurement an integral part of evaluating processes

Source: Bliersbach, C.M., *Guide to Health Care Quality Management*, pp. 7–23, National Association of Quality Assurance Professionals, 1991.

Exhibit 9-4 Joint Commission 10 Step Process Comparison of Quality Assurance
and Quality Improvement

STEP	QUALITY ASSURANCE	QUALITY IMPROVEMENT
1. Responsibility	Assign for monitoring and evaluation activities	Chiefly placed on top management with utilization of interdisciplinary project teams
2. Scope	Limited to clinical departments	All departments of the organization
3. Important Aspects of Care	Monitor high-risk, high-volume, problem-prone areas; not necessarily determined by patient	Important aspects to be determined in collaboration with internal and external customers
4. Indicators	Usually department/program specific	Primarily interdepartmental processes
5. Thresholds	Data points at which further evaluation is triggered	Control limits based on statistical principles
6. Data Collection & Organization	Not specific as to how data should be collected or organized	Accepted statistical methods for collecting and graphing data
7. Evaluation of Care	When thresholds are reached	Seek continuous improvement through reduction of assignable cause or chance cause variation
8. Actions	To improve care or resolve problems	Quality council selects improvement projects according to a formalized selection process
9. Evaluation of Actions	Through continued monitoring of care	Same as QA
10. Communication	Findings, conclusions, recommendations, actions, and results of actions documented and reported through established channels	Same as QA

Source: Bliersbach, C.M., *Guide to Health Care Quality Management,* pp. 7–25, National Association of Quality Assurance Professionals, 1991.

JOINT COMMISSION REQUIREMENTS FOR QUALITY ASSURANCE*

A number of standards for quality assurance are addressed in the accreditation process. The following outline will summarize the points:

- The agency only admits patients whose needs can be met by the services it provides.
- A plan of care is developed and implemented for each patient.
- Care coordination is provided to ensure continuity.
- The patient is appropriately transferred, referred, or discharged.
- Agencies review a sample of records at least quarterly to ensure that records reflect the care provided, condition and progress of the patient, and the condition at discharge.
- There is documented evidence that the patient consents to treatment.
- Services are documented by each person rendering care.
- A plan of treatment is established for every patient.
- Signed orders for treatment are obtained from the physician in a timely manner.
- Staff contacts the physician as needed based on the patient's condition.
- The agency has a process to aid access to consultative services.
- The provision of care demonstrates individualized, goal-directed care.
- The agency has policies and procedures regarding resuscitation.
- Agencies that administer drugs have policies and procedures covering same.
- Personal care and support services are based on initial and ongoing assessment.
- Personal care staff understand duties to be performed.
- Each patient receives care in accordance with the plan of care.

SERVICE AUDITS

An additional type of quality assurance audit differs from the diagnosis-related audit by virtue of its generic nature. This second type, called a service audit, can be applied to any patient who is receiving a specific discipline or service. For example, a home health aide service audit can be applied to any patient receiving this service category regardless of the diagnosis. Another service audit could be physical therapy, and so on.

Like the diagnosis-related audits, these tools should be limited in scope and follow the same process previously discussed. While nursing service audits are

---

*Joint Commission on Accreditation of Healthcare Organizations, *Home Care Standards for Accreditation*, 1991, pp. 7–23.

commercially available, the need for this additional audit is negated by the first part of the diagnosis-related audit, which applies to any patient. It should be reiterated that duplication of audit material is counterproductive. Therefore, this discussion is limited to audits of services exclusive of nursing.

Home Health Aide Service Audit

Most certified agencies have a very large percentage of their visits rendered by home health aides (HHAs). An agency cannot afford to allow this large segment of business to go unmonitored. Now that the Health Care Financing Administration (HCFA) has expanded the coverage to Medicare beneficiaries as a result of court rulings, HHA services can be rendered as often as twice a day, seven days a week, or as needed. The significant growth potential in this service category will necessitate an expanded monitoring role by the quality assurance and improvement committee.

It is recommended that HHAs be allowed to participate in the audit process in the same manner as nurses in accomplishing the diagnosis-related audits, i.e., the aides should complete the audit tool by chart review during a group meeting conducted by the committee, which should offer standby assistance. The completed audits should be validated by selecting a random sample to review to ensure resultant findings are the same. Should audit results be different, reinstruction of the aides would be necessary. The process of aide participation in auditing provides aides with knowledge of the standards by which they are being judged (quality continuation) and helps to reinforce documentation requirements.

A sample audit tool is provided in Exhibit 9–5.

Physical Therapy Service Audit

In agencies that have full-time therapists on staff, the auditing process should be the same as with nurses and aides. Where the agency contracts with therapists to perform visits, it is recommended that the most qualified of these be invited to perform a quarterly review of the service through the appropriate service audit.

The process of physical therapy services should follow the diagram defined in Figure 9–1. An example of a service audit for physical therapy follows (Exhibit 9–6).

Exhibits 9–7 through 9–16 are examples of diagnosis-related audits.

NOTES

1. A. Jacquerye, *The Role of Nursing in Quality Assurance* (Belgium, 1989).
2. B.H. Ente, *Ten Principals of Clinical Indicator Development*.

Exhibit 9–5 Sample Audit Tool 3: Service Audit

SCOPE OF CARE:

Current patients who have received aide services at a frequency of at least twice a week for at least 60 days.

SIGNIFICANT ASPECTS OF CARE:

1. Identifying and reporting changing conditions
2. Personal care rendered

INDICATORS:

1. Structure Indicators: Compliance with aide assignment sheet
2. Process Indicators:
   - Changes called to nurse
   - Changes noted in aide record
3. Outcome Indicators: Established goals achieved and maintained or progress toward goal indicated

THRESHOLDS:

1. Structure Indicators: 95% compliance
2. Process Indicators: 98% compliance
3. Outcome Indicators: 90% compliance

INSTRUCTIONS:

- Check yes when criterion has been met.
- Check no when criterion has not been met.
- Check N/A when criterion does not apply or when the patient's condition changes as a result of an acute episode or document noncompliance.

SERVICE AUDIT OF CERTIFIED NURSING ASSISTANT OR HOME HEALTH AIDE

Client: _____ Date: _____ Branch: _____

Aide Assigned: _____ Client Age: _____ Client Sex: _____

Weekly Visit Frequency: _____

Diagnosis: _____

Functional Limitations: _____

continues

Exhibit 9–5 continued

Possible Points	Actual Points		Yes	No	N/A	Comments
		PART I: Structure Indicator (0 points)				
		1. Does the record indicate any problem with limits on supplies? Data Source: Aide assignment comments section				
		PART II: Process Indicators (70 points)				
		1. Aide assessed, documented, and reported problems to nurse:				
8		a. Vital signs outside of acceptable ranges on assignment sheet				
5		b. Change in skin integrity				
5		c. Change in mental status				
5		d. Subjective changes reported by patient or significant other				
5		e. Change in psychosocial factors				
5		f. Change in environmental factors				
3		g. Change of aide assignment is needed				
3		h. Change of aide weekly visit frequency is needed Data Source: Aide notes last 30 days compared with latest aide assignment				
		2. Aide assessed the need for and gave PRN care and/or documented rationale for not giving PRN care:				
5		a. Mouth care/oral hygiene				
5		b. Hair care/shampoo				
5		c. Nail care/clean and file				
3		d. Assisted with dressing Data Source: Aide notes last two-week period compared with latest aide assignment				

Exhibit 9–5 continued

Possible Points	Actual Points		Yes	No	N/A	Comments
		3. Household duties performed and/or documented rationale for not performing these duties:				
4	_____	a. Bed change/remake				
4	_____	b. Patient's room/bathroom straightened after care given				
5	_____	c. Prepared meals as assigned				
		PART III: Outcome Indicators (30 points)				
10	_____	1. Aide implemented changes as assigned				
10	_____	2. Aide evaluated patient responses to changes in assignment				
10	_____	3. Aide documented goals for patient as being realistic, attainable, unrealistic, unattainable, or met Data Source: Last aide assignment, last week of notes				
100	_____	**TOTALS**				

Remarks: _____

Recommendations: _____

Score: _____   _____
                          Auditor

Possible: 100 Points
No Answers = 0
Example: 80 Points = 80% Compliance Rate

Source: Courtesy of Vickie Trevarthan, RN, Stone Mountain, Georgia.

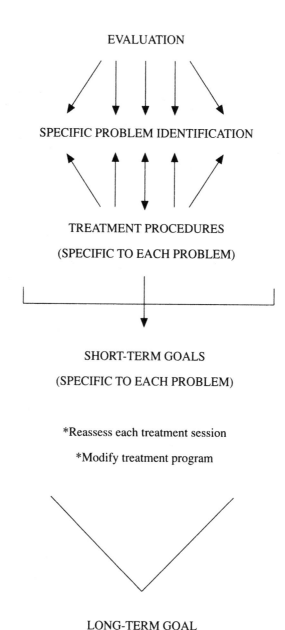

EVALUATION

SPECIFIC PROBLEM IDENTIFICATION

TREATMENT PROCEDURES

(SPECIFIC TO EACH PROBLEM)

SHORT-TERM GOALS

(SPECIFIC TO EACH PROBLEM)

*Reassess each treatment session

*Modify treatment program

LONG-TERM GOAL

OUTCOME IS FINAL FUNCTIONAL RESULT

Figure 9–1 Physical Therapy Service Process. *Source:* Courtesy of Bonnie Blossom, RPT, Roswell, Georgia.

Exhibit 9–6 Sample—Physical Therapy Service Audit

SCOPE OF CARE:

Current patients who have received physical therapy during the last 60 days.

SIGNIFICANT ASPECTS OF CARE:

1. Problem identification
2. Establishment of achievable and measurable goals

INDICATORS:

1. Structure Indicators: Legible documentation, architectural barriers and adaptive equipment, presence or absence of significant other(s)
2. Process Indicators: Problem identification, selection of treatment procedures, establishment of goals, ongoing assessment
3. Outcome Indicators: Use of objective measurement in determining progress, modification of treatment program and goals, communication with other care providers

THRESHOLDS:

1. Structure Indicators: 90% compliance
2. Process Indicators: 98% compliance
3. Outcome Indicators: 95% compliance

Patient _____ Date of Audit _____ Branch _____

Agency Admission Date _____ Client Age _____ Client Sex _____

Start of Patient Care _____ Discharge Therapist _____

Patient Diagnosis _____ Date of Onset _____

Other Pertinent Diagnosis _____ Date of Onset _____

Functional Limitations _____

Possible Points	*Actual Points*		Yes	No	N/A	Comments
		PART I: Structure Indicators (25 points)				
5	_____	1. Registered physical therapist (RPT) assessed the need for safety, adaptive devices, equipment?				
10	_____	2. RPT arranged for devices, equipment, etc.? Data Source: First three visit notes				

continues

Exhibit 9–6 continued

Possible Points	Actual Points		Yes	No	N/A	Comments
10	_____	3. RPT taught rehabilitation program to patient and/or significant others? Data Source: First two weeks of visit notes				
		PART II: Process Indicators (50 points)				
10	_____	1. RPT relates the modalities to the identified problem(s)?				
10	_____	2. RPT uses objective measure to show progress?				
8	_____	3. RPT does continuing assessment of patient's condition and reaction to modalities?				
8	_____	4. RPT modalities and goals are changed in accordance with assessment?				
6	_____	5. RPT implemented changes in treatment modalities?				
8	_____	6. RPT evaluated response to change of modalities? Data Source: Previous 30 days of visit notes				
		PART III: Outcome Indicators (25 points)				
15	_____	1. Are all goals stated in measurable terms? Data Source: Physical therapy assessment/updates				
5	_____	2. RPT checks vital signs (BP, P, R)* every visit?				
5	_____	3. Record reflects RPT is reporting changes in patient's status to the nurse? Data Source: Previous 30 days' notes				

Remarks: _____

Exhibit 9–6 continued

Recommendations: _____
_____
_____

Score:_____   Auditor
Possible: 100 points
All yes & N/A = points
No answers = 0
Example: 80 points = 80% compliance rate

*BP = blood pressure; P = pulse; R = respiration.

Source: Courtesy of Bonnie Blossom, RPT, Roswell, Georgia.

Exhibit 9–7 Sample—Diagnosis-Related Audit for Hypertension

SCOPE OF CARE:

- Primary diagnosis of hypertension newly diagnosed or acute exacerbation
- Patient has been receiving services for at least 30 days

SIGNIFICANT ASPECTS OF CARE:

1. Teaching process
2. Assessment process

CLINICAL INDICATORS:

1. Structure Indicators: Compliance with protocols outside the nurse's control
2. Process Indicators: Compliance with protocols within the nurse's control
3. Outcome Indicators: Result of indicators and patient compliance

THRESHOLDS (evaluation of clinical indicators):

1. Structure Indicators: 85% compliance
2. Process Indicators: 98% compliance
3. Outcome Indicators: 80% compliance

INSTRUCTIONS:

- Check yes when criterion has been met.
- Check no when criterion was not met.
- Check N/A when the criterion does not apply to the patient or when the patient's primary diagnosis changes as a result of an acute episode or document noncompliance. Surveyors are instructed to reduce the points allocated to N/A questions for threshold compliance.

continues

Exhibit 9–7 continued

Possible Points	Actual Points		Yes	No	N/A	Comments
		PART I: Structure Indicators (66 points)				
5		1. Does the record indicate that teaching was directed to the primary caregiver? Data Source: First seven visit notes				
10		2. Are contents of home health aide (HHA) assignments individualized? Data Source: Last HHA assignment sheet				
9		3. Were safety measures identified diagnosis related? Data Source: Plan of treatment (POT)/psycho-social factors				
8		4. Is patient history reflective of primary diagnosis? Data Source: Nurse assessment (history)				
10		5. Are the goals related to the primary diagnosis?				
4		a. Are the stated goals measurable?				
4		b. Are they stated with a time frame? Data Source: POT				
6		6. Is equipment identified? Data Source: Psychosocial factors of RN assessment				
10		7. Is care plan reflective of primary diagnosis?				

Total
Points:
66 _____   Thresholds:
  85% _____

Possible Points	Actual Points		Yes	No	N/A	Comments
		PART II: Process Indicators (243 points)				
		1. Does the record indicate patient or caregiver was taught:				

Exhibit 9–7 continued

Possible Points	Actual Points		Yes	No	N/A	Comments
		a. Nutrition:				
15	_____	i. Diet restriction				
15	_____	ii. Fluid intake				
15	_____	b. Weight monitoring (gain/loss as desirable)				
		c. Medications:				
15	_____	i. Schedule				
15	_____	ii. Actions				
15	_____	iii. Side effects				
15	_____	d. Signs/symptoms of hypertension				
14	_____	e. Signs/symptoms of electrolyte imbalance				
13	_____	f. Signs/symptoms of decreased renal status				
		g. Blood pressure:				
12	_____	i. How to monitor postural blood pressure (sitting, standing, lying)				
12	_____	ii. How to record blood pressure readings				
14	_____	iii. What to report				
10	_____	h. Emergency measures				
10	_____	i. Activity to promote circulation				
10	_____	j. Other complications Data Source: First 30 days of service nurse's notes except emergency measures, which should be on first visit note				
15	_____	2. Were identified safety measures taught? Data Source: Nurse's notes first seven visits				
8	_____	3. Was equipment used checked for safety? Data Source: Psychosocial factors				
20	_____	4. Was care plan updated with pertinent changes and with dates and initials?				

Total
Points: Thresholds:
243 _____   98% _____ _____

continues

Exhibit 9–7 continued

Possible Points	Actual Points		Yes	No	N/A	Comments
		PART III: Outcome Indicators (262 points)				
		1. Does the record indicate:				
		a. Patient or caregiver verbalizes understanding of medication teaching:				
5		i. Schedule				
5		ii. Actions				
5		iii. Side effects				
5		iv. Compliance				
		Data Source: Nurse's notes				
		b. Patient or caregiver verbalizes understanding of:				
5		i. Diet				
5		ii. Fluid intake				
5		iii. Compliance				
		Data Source: Nurse's notes				
14		c. Weight is stable +/– 2 pounds, unless weight gain or loss desirable				
		Data Source: Nurse's notes				
		d. Patient or caregiver verbalizes understanding of:				
12		i. Signs/symptoms of hypertension				
12		ii. Signs/symptoms of electrolyte imbalance				
12		iii. Signs/symptoms of decreased renal status				
		Data Source: Nurse's notes				
14		e. Patient or caregiver verbalizes understanding of emergency measures				
		Data Source: Nurse's notes				
12		f. Edema absent				
10		g. Chest sounds—good expansion with no rales or rhonchi				
8		h. Skin color without pallor or flushing				
		Data Source: Nurse's notes				
		i. Lab values:				
13		i. BUN—10–20 mg/dL				

Exhibit 9–7 continued

Possible Points	Actual Points		Yes	No	N/A	Comments
13	_____	ii. Creatinine—1–1.5 mg/dL				
13	_____	iii. Sodium—136–145 mEq/L				
13	_____	iv. Potassium—3.5–5.0 mEq/L				
		Data Source: Lab results				
		2. Does the record indicate (unless physician orders are evident with specific parameters to the contrary):				
		a. Blood pressure:				
15	_____	i. Sitting—90–140/ 60–90 mm Hg adults less than 50 years				
15	_____	ii. Standing—90–160/ 60–90 mm Hg adults older than 50 years				
15	_____	iii. Lying—Variance less than 20 mm Hg systolic between like extremities sitting/ standing/lying and over a period of time				
		Data Source: Nurse's notes				
13	_____	b. Pulse 60–90 beats per minute and regular				
13	_____	c. Respiratory rate 12–24 breaths per minute at rest and unlabored				
10	_____	d. Temperature is 96.4–99°F orally				
		Data Source: Nurse's notes				

Instructions to #2: If vital signs are outside of stated parameters, the auditor may still give points if the record indicates the nurse noted the change, recorded an explanation, and intervened with notification to the physician.

Total Points: 262 _____

Thresholds: 80% _____

Source: Courtesy of Vickie Trevarthan, RN, Stone Mountain, Georgia.

Exhibit 9–8 Sample—Diagnosis-Related Audit for Cerebrovascular Accident

SCOPE OF CARE:

- Primary diagnosis of cerebrovascular accident (CVA) newly diagnosed
- Patient has been receiving services for at least 60 days

SIGNIFICANT ASPECTS OF CARE:

1. Teaching process
2. Assessment process

CLINICAL INDICATORS:

1. Structure Indicators: Compliance with protocols outside the nurse's control
2. Process Indicators: Compliance with protocols within the nurse's control
3. Outcome Indicators: Result of indicators and patient compliance

THRESHOLDS (evaluation of clinical indicators):

1. Structure Indicators: 85% compliance
2. Process Indicators: 98% compliance
3. Outcome Indicators: 80% compliance

INSTRUCTIONS:

- Check yes when criterion has been met.
- Check no when criterion was not met.
- Check N/A when the criterion does not apply to the patient or when the patient's primary diagnosis changes as a result of an acute episode or document noncompliance. Surveyors are instructed to reduce the points allocated to N/A questions for threshold compliance.

Possible Points	Actual Points		Yes	No	N/A	Comments
		PART I: Structure Indicators (66 points)				
5	_____	1. Does the record indicate that teaching was directed to the primary caregiver? Data Source: First seven visit notes				
10	_____	2. Are contents of home health aide assignments individualized? Data Source: Plan of treatment (POT)/ psychosocial factors				

Exhibit 9–8 continued

Possible Points	Actual Points		Yes	No	N/A	Comments
9	___	3. Were safety measures identified as indicative of diagnosis? Data Source: POT/ psychosocial factors				
8	___	4. Is patient history reflective of primary diagnosis? Data Source: Nurse assessment (history)				
10	___	5. Are the goals related to the primary diagnosis?				
4	___	a. Are the stated goals measurable?				
4	___	b. Are they stated within a time frame?				
6	___	6. Is equipment identified? Data Source: Psychosocial factors of RN assessment				
10	___	7. Is care plan reflective of primary diagnosis?				

Total
Points:
66 ___

Thresholds:
85% ___

Possible Points	Actual Points		Yes	No	N/A	Comments
		PART II: Process Indicators (207 points)				
		1. Does the record indicate patient or caregiver was taught:				
15	___	a. Signs/symptoms of CVA				
		b. Medications:				
5	___	i. Schedule				
5	___	ii. Actions				
5	___	iii. Side effects				
13	___	c. Diet restrictions				
12	___	d. Hydration (1500–2000 mL/day, unless restricted)				
12	___	e. Activities of daily living (ADL)/activity to promote circulation				

continues

Exhibit 9–8 continued

Possible Points	Actual Points		Yes	No	N/A	Comments
12		f. ADL/activity with adaptive devices (if needed)				
13		g. Effective bowel program (if needed)				
13		h. Effective bladder program (if needed)				
11		i. Other complications				
14		j. Emergency measures				
11		k. Prevention of deformities and loss of range of motion (if receiving physical or occupational therapy, mark N/A)				
12		l. Seizure activity and precautions				
11		m. Importance of communication (if receiving speech therapy, mark N/A) Data Source: First 60 days of service nurse's notes except emergency measures, which should be on first visit note				
15		2. Were identified safety measures taught? Data Source: Nurse's notes first seven visits				
8		3. Was equipment used checked for safety? Data Source: Psychosocial factors				
20		4. Was care plan updated with pertinent changes and with dates and initials?				

Total
Points: Thresholds:
207 ____   98% ____

Exhibit 9–8 continued

Possible Points	Actual Points		Yes	No	N/A	Comments
		PART III: Outcome Indicators (270 points)				
15	_____	1. Patient or caregiver verbalizes understanding of signs and symptoms of CVA				
15	_____	2. Patient or caregiver knows what to report to physician				
		3. Patient or caregiver verbalizes understanding of medication teaching:				
5	_____	a. Schedule (drug, dosage, route, and time)				
5	_____	b. Actions				
5	_____	c. Side effects				
5	_____	d. Compliance				
12	_____	4. Weight stable +/− 2 pounds (unless gain or loss desirable)				
12	_____	5. Record indicates patient is hydrated				
4	_____	6. Symptoms none or controlled:				
4	_____	a. Edema				
4	_____	b. Vertigo				
4	_____	c. Headaches				
4	_____	d. Fainting				
12	_____	7. Dyspnea none				
12	_____	8. Chest sounds clear				
12	_____	9. Skin color is without pallor or flushing				
13	_____	10. Bowel program is effective				
13	_____	11. Bladder program is effective				
14	_____	12. Patient or caregiver verbalizes understanding of emergency measures				
13	_____	13. Record indicates patient's activities of daily living independence/dependence corresponds to limitations				
14	_____	14. Patient or caregiver verbalizes understanding of seizure activity and precautions				

continues

Exhibit 9–8 continued

Possible Points	Actual Points		Yes	No	N/A	Comments
11	_____	15. Patient has not developed deformities, contractures, or loss of range of motion (if receiving physical or occupational therapy, mark N/A)				
11	_____	16. Patient has effective method of communicating (if receiving speech therapy, mark N/A)				
		17. Does the record indicate that (unless physician orders are evident with specific parameters to the contrary):				
15	_____	a. Blood pressure is maintained between 90/60–160/90 mm Hg				
12	_____	b. Pulse is 60–90 beats per minute and regular				
12	_____	c. Respiratory rate is 12–24 breaths per minute at rest and unlabored				
12	_____	d. Temperature is 96.4–99°F orally				

Data Source: Plan of treatment

Instructions to #17: If vital signs are outside of stated parameters, the auditor may still give points if the record indicates the nurse noted the change, recorded an explanation, and intervened with notification to the physician.

Total Points: 270 _____   Thresholds: 80% _____

Source: Courtesy of Vickie Trevarthan, RN, Stone Mountain, Georgia.

Exhibit 9–9 Sample—Diagnosis-Related Audit for Congestive Heart Failure

---

SCOPE OF CARE:

- Congestive heart failure (CHF) new onset or acute exacerbation (primary diagnosis)
- Patient has been receiving services for at least 30 days

SIGNIFICANT ASPECTS OF CARE:

1. Teaching process
2. Assessment process

CLINICAL INDICATORS:

1. Structure Indicators: Compliance with protocols outside the nurse's control
2. Process Indicators: Compliance with protocols within the nurse's control
3. Outcome Indicators: Result of indicators and patient compliance

THRESHOLDS (evaluation of clinical indicators):

1. Structure Indicators: 85% compliance
2. Process Indicators: 98% compliance
3. Outcome Indicators: 80% compliance

INSTRUCTIONS:

- Check yes when criterion has been met.
- Check no when criterion was not met.
- Check N/A when the criterion does not apply to the patient or when the patient's primary diagnosis changes as a result of an acute episode or document noncompliance. Surveyors are instructed to reduce the points allocated to N/A questions for threshold compliance.

Possible Points	*Actual Points*		Yes	No	N/A	Comments
		PART I: Structure Indicators (66 points)				
5	_____	1. Does the record indicate that teaching was directed to the primary caregiver? Data Source: First seven visit notes				
10	_____	2. Are contents of home health aide (HHA) assignments individualized? Data Source: Last HHA assignment sheet				

continues

Exhibit 9–9 continued

Possible Points	Actual Points		Yes	No	N/A	Comments
9		3. Were safety measures identified as indicative of diagnosis? Data Source: Plan of treatment (POT)/ psychosocial factors				
8		4. Is patient history reflective of primary diagnosis? Data Source: Nurse assessment (history)				
10		5. Are the goals related to the primary diagnosis?				
4		a. Are the stated goals measurable?				
4		b. Are they stated with a time frame? Data Source: POT				
6		6. Is equipment identified? Data Source: Psychosocial factors of RN assessment				
10		7. Is care plan reflective of primary diagnosis?				

Total Points
66 _____   Thresholds:
85% _____ _____

Possible Points	Actual Points		Yes	No	N/A	Comments
		PART II: Process Indicators (196 points) 1. Does the record indicate patient or caregiver was taught:				
15		a. Signs/symptoms of CHF				
12		b. Diet management				
12		c. Fluid restriction				
6		d. i. How to take pulse				
6		ii. Knows what to report				
6		e. i. Frequency to check weight				
6		ii. Process for monitoring weight				

Exhibit 9–9 continued

Possible Points	Actual Points		Yes	No	N/A	Comments
		f. Medications:				
10		i. Schedule				
10		ii. Actions				
10		iii. Side effects				
14		g. Emergency measures				
14		h. Oxygen precautions				
8		i. Activity level and/or restrictions				
8		j. Circulatory enhancement				
8		k. Signs/symptoms of electrolyte imbalance				
8		l. Other complications Data Source: First 30 days of service nurse's notes, except emergency measures, which should be on first visit note				
15		2. Were identified safety measures taught? Data Source: Nurse's notes first seven visits				
8		3. Was equipment used checked for safety? Data Source: Psychosocial factors				
20		4. Was care plan updated with pertinent changes and with dates and initials?				

Total Points
196 ___

Thresholds:
98% ___

Possible Points	Actual Points		Yes	No	N/A	Comments
		PART III: Outcome Indicators (267 points)				
		1. Does the record indicate:				
15		a. Patient is able to pace activity without dyspnea on exertion (DOE)/ shortness of breath (SOB) Data Source: Nurse's notes				

continues

Exhibit 9–9 continued

Possible Points	Actual Points		Yes	No	N/A	Comments
15	_____	b. Chest sounds clear without rales or rhonchi Data Source: Nurse's notes				
14	_____	c. Lung function—No dyspnea on exertion (DOE)/SOB; dyspnea controlled Data Source: Nurse's notes				
13	_____	d. Cyanosis—None Data Source: Nurse's notes				
5	_____	e. Patient or caregiver verbalizes understanding of:				
5	_____	i. Diet				
5	_____	ii. Fluid restriction				
5	_____	iii. Compliance Data Source: Nurse's notes				
15	_____	f. Weight stable +/− 2 pounds, unless weight gain or loss desirable Data Source: Nurse's notes				
10	_____	g. Nausea, vomiting, anorexia—None Data Source: Nurse's notes				
		h. Patient or caregiver verbalizes understanding of medication teaching:				
5	_____	i. Schedule (drug, dosage, route, and time)				
5	_____	ii. Actions				
5	_____	iii. Side effects				
5	_____	iv. Compliance Data Source: Nurse's notes				
		i. Lab values:				
10	_____	i. Sodium—135–145 mEq/L				
14	_____	ii. Potassium—3.5–5.3 MEq/L				

Exhibit 9-9 continued

Possible Points	Actual Points		Yes	No	N/A	Comments
14	___	iii. Digoxin level—0.5–2.0 Ng/mL Data Source: Lab results				
		j. Patient or caregiver verbalizes understanding of:				
12	___	i. Signs/symptoms of congestive heart failure				
12	___	ii. Signs/symptoms of toxicity				
12	___	iii. Signs/symptoms of electrolyte imbalance				
14	___	k. Patient or caregiver verbalizes understanding of emergency measures.				
		2. Does the record indicate that (unless physician orders are evident with specific parameters to the contrary):				
14	___	a. Blood pressure is maintained between 90/60–160/90 mm Hg				
15	___	b. Pulse is 60–90 beats per minute and regular				
14	___	c. Respiratory rate is 12–24 breaths per minute at rest and unlabored				
14	___	d. Temperature is 96.4–99°F orally Data Source: Nurse's notes				

Instructions to #2: If vital signs are outside of stated parameters, the auditor may still give points if the record indicates the nurse noted the change, recorded an explanation and intervened with notification to the physician.

Total points		Thresholds:	
267	___	80%	___

Source: Courtesy of Vickie Trevarthan, RN, Stone Mountain, Georgia.

Exhibit 9–10 Sample—Diagnosis-Related Audit for Chronic Obstructive Pulmonary Disease

---

SCOPE OF CARE:

• Chronic obstructive pulmonary disease (COPD) new onset or acute exacerbation (primary diagnosis)
• Patient has been receiving services for at least 30 days

SIGNIFICANT ASPECTS OF CARE:

1. Teaching process
2. Assessment process

CLINICAL INDICATORS:

1. Structure Indicators: Compliance with protocols outside the nurse's control
2. Process Indicators: Compliance with protocols within the nurse's control
3. Outcome Indicators: Result of indicators and patient compliance

THRESHOLDS (evaluation of clinical indicators):

1. Structure Indicators: 85% compliance
2. Process Indicators: 98% compliance
3. Outcome Indicators: 80% compliance

INSTRUCTIONS:

• Check yes when criterion has been met.
• Check no when criterion was not met.
• Check N/A when the criterion does not apply to the patient or when the patient's primary diagnosis changes as a result of an acute episode or document noncompliance. Surveyors are instructed to reduce the points allocated to N/A questions for threshold compliance.

Possible Points	Actual Points		Yes	No	N/A	Comments
		PART I: Structure Indicators (66 points)				
5	_____	1. Does the record indicate that teaching was directed to the primary caregiver? Data Source: First seven visit notes				
10	_____	2. Are contents of home health aide (HHA) assignments individualized? Data Source: Last HHA assignment sheet				

Exhibit 9–10 continued

Possible Points	Actual Points		Yes	No	N/A	Comments
9	_____	3. Were safety measures identified as indicative of diagnosis? Data Source: Plan of treatment/psychosocial factors				
8	_____	4. Is patient history reflective of primary diagnosis? Data Source: Nurse assessment (history)				
10	_____	5. Are the goals related to the primary diagnosis?				
4	_____	a. Are the stated goals measurable?				
4	_____	b. Are they stated with a time frame? Data Source: Plan of treatment				
6	_____	6. Is equipment identified? Data Source: Psychosocial factors of RN assessment				
10	_____	7. Is care plan reflective of primary diagnosis?				

Total Points: 66	_____	Thresholds: 85% _____

Possible Points	Actual Points		Yes	No	N/A	Comments
		PART II: Process Indicators (240 points) 1. Does the record indicate patient or caregiver was taught signs/symptoms of chronic obstructive pulmonary disease (COPD):				
5	_____	a. Medications:				
5	_____	i. Schedule				
5	_____	ii. Actions				
5	_____	iii. Side effects				
15	_____	b. Oxygen usage per order				
14	_____	c. Infection control measures with use of oxygen				

continues

Exhibit 9–10 continued

Possible Points	Actual Points		Yes	No	N/A	Comments
14	___	d. Respiration exercises				
		e. Sputum management:				
14	___	i. Effective cough technique				
13	___	ii. Postural drainage (if ordered)				
13	___	iii. Clapping (if ordered)				
14	___	f. Productive cough				
11	___	g. Effects of respiratory irritants				
12	___	h. Activities of daily living organization around shortness of breath needed for oxygen				
13	___	i. Hydration of 2000 mL/ day (unless restricted)				
12	___	j. Well-balanced diet with small frequent feedings (if necessary)				
10	___	k. Other complications				
14	___	l. Emergency measures Data Source: First 30 days of service nurse's notes, except emergency measures, which should be on first visit note				
15	___	2. Were identified safety measures taught? Data Source: Nurse's notes first seven visits				
16	___	3. Was equipment used checked for safety? Data Source: Psychosocial factors				
20	___	4. Was care plan updated with pertinent changes and with dates and initials?				

Total
Points:
240   ___   Thresholds:
                 98%   ___

Exhibit 9–10 continued

Possible Points	Actual Points		Yes	No	N/A	Comments
		PART III: Outcome Indicators (244 points)				
		1. Does the record indicate:				
		a. Patient or caregiver verbalizes understanding of medication teaching:				
5		i. Schedule				
5		ii. Actions				
5		iii. Side effects				
5		iv. Compliance				
		b. Patient or caregiver verbalizes understanding of:				
10		i. Emergency measures				
10		ii. Oxygen usage per order				
10		iii. Infection control measures with use of oxygen				
9		iv. Avoidance of respiratory irritants				
15		c. Patient is well hydrated				
15		d. No dyspnea at rest				
10		e. Chest sounds clear without rales or rhonchi				
15		f. Sputum is colorless, white, or clear				
10		g. No chest pain				
9		h. Optimal weight stable +/− 2 pounds				
7		i. No edema				
12		j. Free of other complications (upper respiratory infection (URI), congestive heart failure (CHF), cardiac arrhythmias, thrombosis)				
		Data Source: Nurse's notes				
		k. Does the record indicate lab values:				
10		i. Blood gases— PcO_2 35–45 mm Hg PO_2 80–90 mm Hg				

continues

Exhibit 9–10 continued

Possible Points	Actual Points		Yes	No	N/A	Comments
		(Lab values done either per physician, skilled nurse (SN), or durable medical equipment (DME) if using pulse oximetry reading. Greater than 90 saturation is a normal reading. If reading is not within this range the physician is made aware and given acceptable reading for client.)				
10	___	ii. Theophylline levels—10–20 µg/mL (If patient is on other bronchodilators, lab values are to be within normal limits—or have an order that physician is aware and approves levels.) Data Source: Lab results				
15	___	2. Does the record indicate that (unless physician orders are evident with specific parameters to the contrary):				
13	___	a. Blood pressure is maintained between 90/60–160/90 mm Hg				
15	___	b. Pulse is 60–90 beats per minute and regular				
15	___	c. Respiration—good chest expansion without hyperextension/not labored/quiet; rate 12–24 breaths per minute at rest				
14	___	d. Temperature is 96.4–99°F orally Data Source: Nurse's notes				

Exhibit 9–10 continued

Possible Points	*Actual Points*	
		Instructions to #2: If vital signs are outside of stated parameters, the auditor may still give points if the record indicates the nurse noted the change, recorded an explanation, and intervened with notification to the physician.

Total
Points: Thresholds:
244   80%

Source: Courtesy of Vickie Trevarthan, RN, Stone Mountain, Georgia.

Exhibit 9–11 Sample—Diagnosis-Related Audit for Atonic Bladder

SCOPE OF CARE:

- Atonic bladder (primary diagnosis)
- Patient has been receiving services for at least 90 days

SIGNIFICANT ASPECTS OF CARE:

1. Teaching process
2. Assessment process
3. Treatment protocol

CLINICAL INDICATORS:

1. Structure Indicators: Compliance with protocols outside the nurse's control
2. Process Indicators: Compliance with protocols within the nurse's control
3. Outcome Indicators: Result of indicators and patient compliance

THRESHOLDS (evaluation of clinical indicators):

1. Structure Indicators: 85% compliance
2. Process Indicators: 98% compliance
3. Outcome Indicators: 80% compliance

continues

Exhibit 9–11 continued

INSTRUCTIONS:

- Check yes when criterion has been met.
- Check no when criterion was not met.
- Check N/A when the criterion does not apply to the patient or when the patient's primary diagnosis changes as a result of an acute episode or document noncompliance. Surveyors are instructed to reduce the points allocated to N/A questions for threshold compliance.

Possible Points	Actual Points		Yes	No	N/A	Comments
		PART I: Structure Indicators (66 points)				
5		1. Does the record indicate that teaching was directed to the primary caregiver? Data Source: First seven visit notes				
10		2. Are contents of home health aide (HHA) assignments individualized? Data Source: Last HHA assignment sheet				
9		3. Were identified safety measures diagnosis related? Data Source: Plan of treatment/psychosocial factors				
8		4. Is patient history reflective of primary diagnosis? Data Source: Nurse assessment (history)				
10		5. Are the goals related to the primary diagnosis?				
4		a. Are the stated goals measurable?				
4		b. Are they stated with a time frame? Data Source: Plan of treatment				
6		6. Is equipment identified? Data Source: Psychosocial factors of RN assessment				
10		7. Is care plan reflective of primary diagnosis?				

Total Points: 66 _____

Thresholds: 85% _____

Exhibit 9-11 continued

Possible Points	Actual Points		Yes	No	N/A	Comments
		PART II: Process Indicators (360 points)				
		1. Does the record indicate patient or caregiver was taught:				
		a. Fluid intake				
15		i. 3 or more liters a day, unless contraindicated				
13		ii. Recording fluid intake				
13		b. Balanced diet, unless otherwise ordered				
14		c. Signs/symptoms of urinary tract infection				
14		d. What to report to physician/nurse				
		e. Care of closed urinary system:				
14		i. Positioning				
14		ii. Emptying				
14		iii. Catheter care including frequency and with what, i.e., soap and water, etc.				
14		iv. Removal of catheter if it becomes plugged				
		f. Catheter irrigation, if applicable:				
14		i. Rationale for catheter irrigation				
14		ii. Type of solution				
14		iii. Amount of solution				
14		iv. Frequency of irrigation				
14		g. How to change urinary drainage bag to leg bag if used				
		h. Infection control precautions with:				
14		i. Manipulation of urinary system				
14		ii. Disposal of urine				
14		iii. Cleaning and storage of urinary collection container				

continues

Exhibit 9–11 continued

Possible Points	Actual Points		Yes	No	N/A	Comments
14	___	iv. Proper usage of irrigation kit				
14	___	v. Proper handling of irrigation solution				
		i. Medications:				
14	___	i. Schedule (drug, dosage, route, and time)				
13	___	ii. Actions				
13	___	iii. Side effects				
12	___	j. Other complications Data Source: First 30 days of service nurse's notes except emergency measures, which should be on first visit note				
15	___	2. Were identified safety measures taught? Data Source: Nurse's notes first seven visits				
8	___	3. Was equipment used checked for safety? Data Source: Psychosocial factors				
20	___	4. Was care plan updated with pertinent changes and with dates and initials?				

Total Points: 360 ___   Thresholds: 98% ___

Possible Points	Actual Points		Yes	No	N/A	Comments
		PART III: Outcome Indicators (368 points)				
		1. Does the record indicate:				
15	___	a. Patient is hydrated				
13	___	b. Weight stable +/– 2 pounds unless weight gain or loss is indicated				
14	___	c. Asymptomatic/free from urinary tract infection Data Source: Nurse's notes or lab results				

Exhibit 9–11 continued

Possible Points	Actual Points		Yes	No	N/A	Comments
13		d. Patient or caregiver verbalizes understanding of what to report to physician/nurse				
		e. Patient or caregiver demonstrates care of closed urinary system:				
14		i. Positioning				
14		ii. Emptying				
14		iii. Catheter care				
14		iv. Removal of catheter				
13		f. Patient or caregiver verbalizes understanding of why catheter irrigation is needed				
13		g. Patient or caregiver demonstrates catheter irrigation (if applicable)				
14		i. With use of correct irrigating solution				
14		ii. With use of correct amount of irrigating solution				
14		h. Patient or caregiver verbalizes correct catheter irrigation frequency per order				
14		i. Patient or caregiver demonstrates proper technique of changing urinary drainage bag if using leg bag				
		j. Patient or caregiver demonstrates infection control precautions:				
14		i. Any manipulation of urinary system				
14		ii. Disposal of urine				
14		iii. Proper care of collection container				
14		iv. Proper care of irrigation solution				
14		v. Proper care of irrigation kit				

continues

Exhibit 9–11 continued

Possible Points	Actual Points		Yes	No	N/A	Comments
		k. Patient or caregiver verbalizes understanding of medication teaching:				
14		i. Schedule				
13		ii. Actions				
13		iii. Side effects				
14		iv Compliance				
		2. Does the record indicate that (unless physician orders are evident with specific parameters to the contrary):				
12		a. Blood pressure is maintained between 90/60–160/90 mm Hg				
12		b. Pulse is 60–90 beats per minute and regular				
12		c. Respiratory rate is 12–24 breaths per minute at rest and unlabored				
15		d. Temperature is 96.4–99°F orally				
		Data Source: Nurse's notes				

Instructions to #2: If vital signs are outside of stated parameters, the auditor may still give points if the record indicates the nurse noted the change, recorded an explanation, and intervened with notification to the physician.

Total Points: 368

Thresholds: 80%

Source: Courtesy of Vickie Trevarthan, RN, Stone Mountain, Georgia.

Exhibit 9–12 Sample—Diagnosis-Related Audit for Failure To Thrive

SCOPE OF CARE:

- Failure to thrive (primary diagnosis)
- Appropriate for gestational age
- Patient has been receiving services for at least 60 days

SIGNIFICANT ASPECTS OF CARE:

1. Teaching process
2. Assessment process

CLINICAL INDICATORS:

1. Structure Indicators: Compliance with protocols outside the nurse's control
2. Process Indicators: Compliance with protocols within the nurse's control
3. Outcome Indicators: Result of indicators and patient compliance

THRESHOLDS (evaluation of clinical indicators):

1. Structure Indicators: 85% compliance
2. Process Indicators: 98% compliance
3. Outcome Indicators: 80% compliance

INSTRUCTIONS:

- Check yes when criterion has been met.
- Check no when criterion was not met.
- Check N/A when the criterion does not apply to the patient or when the patient's primary diagnosis changes as a result of an acute episode or document noncompliance. Surveyors are instructed to reduce the points allocated to N/A questions for threshold compliance.

Possible Points	Actual Points		Yes	No	N/A	Comments
		PART I: Structure Indicators (56 points)				
5	_____	1. Does the record indicate that teaching was directed to the primary caregiver? Data Source: First seven visit notes				
9	_____	2. Were safety measures identified as indicative of diagnosis? Data Source: Plan of treatment/ psychosocial factors				

continues

Exhibit 9–12 continued

Possible Points	Actual Points		Yes	No	N/A	Comments
8		3. Is patient history reflective of primary diagnosis? Data Source: Nurse assessment (history)				
10		4. Are the goals related to the primary diagnosis?				
4		a. Are the stated goals measurable?				
4		b. Are they stated with a time frame? Data Source: Plan of treatment				
6		5. Is equipment identified? Data Source: Psychosocial factors of RN assessment				
10		6. Is care plan reflective of primary diagnosis?				

Total Points: 56

Thresholds: 85%

Possible Points	Actual Points		Yes	No	N/A	Comments
		PART II: Process Indicators (233 points) 1. Does the record indicate nurse assessed:				
10		a. Previous feeding patterns Data Source: Nursing assessment				
10		b. Maternal-infant bonding Data Source: Nursing assessment and/or first seven visit notes				
10		c. Growth pattern Data Source: Growth chart				
10		d. Developmental parameters Data Source: Denver Developmental Screening Test (DDST)				

Exhibit 9–12 continued

Possible Points	Actual Points		Yes	No	N/A	Comments
		e. Sensory:				
5		i. Visual				
5		ii. Hearing				
		Data Source: Nursing assessment				
		2. Does the record indicate caregiver was taught:				
10		a. Feeding techniques				
15		b. Positioning after feedings				
10		c. Infant stimulation				
10		d. Anticipatory guidance				
15		e. Infancy cardiopulmonary resuscitation (CPR)				
15		f. Emergency measures				
		Data Source: Nurse's notes on first visit				
15		g. Signs and symptoms of illness				
10		h. Well baby care				
10		i. Bathing technique				
10		j. Checking axillary temperature				
15		k. What to report to physician				
10		l. Utilization of appropriate community resources				
		Data Source: First 60 days of service nurse's notes except emergency measures, which should be on first visit note				
10		3. Were identified safety measures taught?				
		Data Source: Nurse's notes first seven visits				
8		4. Was equipment used checked for safety?				
		Data Source: Psychosocial factors				
20		5. Was care plan updated with pertinent changes and with dates and initials?				

continues

Exhibit 9–12 continued

Total Points: 243		Thresholds: 98%				

Possible Points	Actual Points		Yes	No	N/A	Comments
		PART III: Outcome Indicators (219 points)				
		1. Does the record indicate:				
20		a. Growth maintained on appropriate curve Data Source: Growth chart				
20		b. Maternal-infant bonding Data Source: Nurse's notes				
18		c. Retesting of developmental parameters indicates they are within normal limits Data Source: DDST				
20		d. Caregiver verbalizes signs of illness				
20		e. Caregiver verbalizes understanding of infant CPR				
20		f. Caregiver verbalizes understanding of well baby care				
20		g. Caregiver verbalizes what to report to physician				
		h. Caregiver demonstrates proper technique for:				
15		i. Bathing baby				
15		ii. Taking axillary temperature				
15		iii. Positioning baby after feedings				
		2. Does the record indicate that (unless physician orders are evident with specific parameters to the contrary):				
12		a. Pulse is 60–200 beats per minute and regular				

Exhibit 9–12 continued

Possible Points	Actual Points		Yes	No	N/A	Comments
12	___	b. Respiratory rate is 20–44 breaths per minute at rest and unlabored				
12	___	c. Temperature is 96–99°F axillary				
___	___	Data Source: Nurse's notes				

Instructions to #2: If vital signs are outside of stated parameters, the auditor may still give points if the record indicates the nurse noted the change, recorded an explanation, and intervened with notification to the physician.

Total
Points: Thresholds:
219 ___   80% ___

Source: Courtesy of Vickie Trevarthan, RN, and Bonnie Dyer, RN.

Exhibit 9–13 Sample—Diangosis-Related Audit for Acquired Immune Deficiency Syndrome

SCOPE OF CARE:

- Acquired immune deficiency syndrome (primary diagnosis)
- Patient has been receiving services for at least 60 days

SIGNIFICANT ASPECTS OF CARE:

1. Teaching process
2. Assessment process
3. Treatment protocols

continues

Exhibit 9–13 continued

CLINICAL INDICATORS:

1. Structure Indicators: Compliance with protocols outside the nurse's control
2. Process Indicators: Compliance with protocols within the nurse's control
3. Outcome Indicators: Result of indicators and patient compliance

THRESHOLDS (evaluation of clinical indicators):

1. Structure Indicators: 85% compliance
2. Process Indicators: 98% compliance
3. Outcome Indicators: 80% compliance

INSTRUCTIONS:

- Check yes when criterion has been met.
- Check no when criterion was not met.
- Check N/A when the criterion does not apply to the patient or when the patient's primary diagnosis changes as a result of an acute episode or document noncompliance. Surveyors are instructed to reduce the points allocated to N/A questions for threshold compliance.

Possible Points	Actual Points		Yes	No	N/A	Comments
		PART I: Structure Indicators (66 points)				
5	____	1. Does the record indicate that teaching was directed to the primary caregiver? Data Source: First seven visit notes				
10	____	2. Are contents of home health aide (HHA) assignments individualized? Data Source: Last HHA assignment sheet				
9	____	3. Were safety measures identified as indicative of diagnosis? Data Source: Plan of treatment/psychosocial factors				
8	____	4. Is patient history reflective of primary diagnosis? Data Source: Nurse assessment (history)				
10	____	5. Are the goals related to the primary diagnosis?				

Exhibit 9–13 continued

Possible Points	Actual Points		Yes	No	N/A	Comments
4	___	a. Are the stated goals measurable?				
4	___	b. Are they stated with a time frame? Data Source: Plan of treatment				
6	___	6. Is equipment identified? Data Source: Psychosocial factors of RN assessment				
10	___	7. Is care plan reflective of primary diagnosis?				

Total Points: 66 ___ Thresholds: 85% ___

Possible Points	Actual Points		Yes	No	N/A	Comments
		PART II: Process Indicators (273 points) 1. Does the record indicate patient or caregiver was taught: a. Medications				
5	___	i. Schedule (drug, dosage, route, and time)				
5	___	ii. Actions				
5	___	iii. Side effects				
5	___	b. Principles of balanced diet: High-calorie, high-protein, high-fiber				
5	___	i. Dietary supplement as ordered for weight gain				
5	___	ii. Fluid intake to maintain hydration				
14	___	c. Signs/symptoms of dehydration				
12	___	d. Importance of meticulous hygiene				
12	___	e. Energy conservation measures				
12	___	f. Signs/symptoms of anxiety				

continues

Exhibit 9–13 continued

Possible Points	Actual Points		Yes	No	N/A	Comments
12	_____	g. Relaxation techniques to ease anxiety				
13	_____	h. Safety precautions when at risk for bleeding				
13	_____	i. Signs/symptoms of bleeding				
14	_____	j. What to report to physician/nurse				
13	_____	k. Preventive skin care— avoid injury to skin or mucous membranes				
13	_____	l. Signs/symptoms of wound infection				
13	_____	m. Pursed-lip, diaphragmatic breathing exercises to decrease respiratory effort required				
15	_____	n. Administration of enterals or parenterals				
15	_____	o. Care of venous access device				
15	_____	p. Infection control precautions at home				
14	_____	q. Signs/symptoms of AIDS-related infections and concerns				
		Data Source: First days of service nurse's notes except emergency measures, which should be on first visit note				
15	_____	2. Were identified safety measures taught? Data Source: Nurse's notes first 7 visits				
8	_____	3. Was equipment used checked for safety? Data Source: Psychosocial factors				
20	_____	4. Was care plan updated with pertinent changes and with dates and initials?				

Exhibit 9–13 continued

Total Points: 273	Thresholds: 98%

Possible Points	Actual Points		Yes	No	N/A	Comments
		PART III: Outcome Indicators (278 points)				
		1. Patient or caregiver verbalizes understanding of medication teaching:				
5		a. Schedule (drug, dosage, route, and time)				
5		b. Actions				
5		c. Side effects				
5		d. Compliance Data Source: Nurse's notes				
15		2. Pain—None/Controlled Data Source: Nurse's notes				
15		3. Weight stable +/– 5 pounds, unless weight gain desirable Data Source: Nurse's notes				
15		4. Hydrated Data Source: Nurse's notes				
15		5. Skin intact, no new areas of skin breakdown since admission to agency Data Source: Nurse's notes				
14		6. Patient or caregiver verbalizes signs and symptoms of wound infection—if applicable Data Source: Nurse's notes				
13		7. Patient or caregiver verbalizes signs and symptoms of anxiety and techniques for relaxation Data Source: Nurse's notes				
15		8. Lab values: Complete blood cell count with differential/sequential multiple analysis (SMA)–22 (within normal limits unless other parameters are approved by physician) Data Source: Lab results				

continues

Exhibit 9–13 continued

Possible Points	Actual Points		Yes	No	N/A	Comments
15		9. Patient or caregiver verbalizes understanding of signs and symptoms of bleeding				
15		10. Patient or caregiver verbalizes understanding of what to report to physician/ nurse				
14		11. Lungs clear without dyspnea on exertion or shortness of breath				
15		12. Patient or caregiver demonstrates correct techniques of administration of enterals or parenterals				
15		13. Patient or caregiver demonstrates care of venous access device				
14		14. Patient or caregiver verbalizes understanding of home infection control precautions				
14		15. Patient or caregiver verbalizes understanding of signs and symptoms of AIDS-related infections and concerns				
		16. Does the record indicate that (unless physician orders are evident with specific parameters to the contrary):				
12		a. Blood pressure is maintained between 90/60–160/90 mm Hg				
12		b. Pulse is 60–90 beats per minute and regular				
15		c. Respiratory rate is 12–24 breaths per minute at rest and unlabored				
15		d. Temperature is 96.4–99°F orally				

Data Source for #9–16:
Nurse's notes

Exhibit 9–13 continued

Possible Points	*Actual Points*	
		Instructions to #16: If vital signs are outside of stated parameters, the auditor may still give points if the record indicates the nurse noted the change, recorded an explanation, and intervened with notification to the physician.
Total Points: 278 _____		Thresholds: 80% _____ _____

Source: Courtesy of Vickie Trevarthan, RN, Stone Mountain, Georgia.

Exhibit 9–14 Sample—Diagnosis-Related Audit for Decubiti/Wounds (Surgical or Trauma)

SCOPE OF CARE:

- Decubiti/wounds (primary diagnosis)
- Patient admitted within 60 days of audit

SIGNIFICANT ASPECTS OF CARE:

1. Treatment protocol
2. Assessment process
3. Teaching process

CLINICAL INDICATORS:

1. Structure Indicators: Compliance with protocols outside the nurse's control
2. Process Indicators: Compliance with protocols within the nurse's control
3. Outcome Indicators: Result of indicators and patient compliance

THRESHOLDS (evaluation of clinical indicators):

1. Structure Indicators: 85% compliance
2. Process Indicators: 98% compliance
3. Outcome Indicators: 80% compliance

continues

Exhibit 9–14 continued

INSTRUCTIONS:

- Check yes when criterion has been met.
- Check no when criterion was not met.
- Check N/A when the criterion does not apply to the patient or when the patient's primary diagnosis changes as a result of an acute episode or document noncompliance. Surveyors are instructed to reduce the points allocated to N/A questions for threshold compliance.

Possible Points	Actual Points		Yes	No	N/A	Comments
		PART I: Structure Indicators (66 points)				
5	___	1. Does the record indicate that teaching was directed to the primary caregiver? Data Source: First seven visit notes				
10	___	2. Are contents of home health aide (HHA) assignments individualized? Data Source: Last HHA assignment sheet				
9	___	3. Were safety measures identified as indicative of diagnosis? Data Source: Plan of treatment/psychosocial factors				
8	___	4. Is patient history reflective of primary diagnosis? Data Source: Nurse assessment (history)				
10	___	5. Are the goals related to the primary diagnosis?				
4	___	a. Are the stated goals measurable?				
4	___	b. Are they stated with a time frame? Data Source: Plan of treatment				
6	___	6. Is equipment identified? Data Source: Psychosocial factors of nurse assessment				
10	___	7. Is care plan reflective of primary diagnosis?				

Total Points:
66   ___

Thresholds:
85%   ___

Exhibit 9–14 continued

Possible Points	Actual Points		Yes	No	N/A	Comments
		PART II: Process Indicators (190 points)				
		1. Does the record indicate patient/caregiver was taught:				
15		a. Signs and symptoms of infection or complications				
15		b. Procedure for wound care/dressing change per aseptic/sterile technique				
14		c. Measures to reduce pressure				
14		d. Measures to enhance circulation				
13		e. Activity to promote healing (within any restrictions)				
		f. Diet of:				
5		i. High protein, unless contraindicated				
5		ii. High carbohydrate, unless contraindicated				
5		iii. High vitamin C, unless contra-indicated				
14		g. Hydration 2+ liters fluid per day, unless contraindicated				
10		h. Emergency measures				
		i. Medications:				
4		i. Schedule				
4		ii. Actions				
4		iii. Side effects				
10		j. Other complications				
		Data Source: First 60 days of service nurse's notes except emergency measures, which should be on first visit note				
15		2. Wound measurements of the week				
15		3. Were identified safety measures taught?				
		Data Source: Nurse's notes first seven visits				

continues

Exhibit 9–14 continued

Possible Points	Actual Points		Yes	No	N/A	Comments
8	_____	4. Was equipment used checked for safety? Data Source: Psychosocial factors				
20	_____	5. Was care plan updated with pertinent changes and with dates and initials?				

Total
Points: Thresholds:
190   _____   98%   _____

Possible Points	Actual Points		Yes	No	N/A	Comments
		PART III: Outcome Indicators (275 points)				
		1. Does the record indicate:				
13	_____	a. Pain none/controlled				
		b. Patient or caregiver verbalizes understanding of:				
4	_____	i. Medication schedule				
4	_____	ii. Actions				
4	_____	iii. Side effects				
4	_____	iv. Compliance				
		c. Patient or caregiver verbalizes understanding of:				
4	_____	i. Dietary needs				
4	_____	ii. Fluid intake				
4	_____	iii. Compliance with diet				
4	_____	iv. Compliance with fluid intake				
13	_____	d. Weight stable +/– 2 pounds, unless weight gain or loss desirable				
14	_____	e. Patient or caregiver verbalizes understanding of signs and symptoms of infection or complications				
15	_____	f. Patient or caregiver demonstrates correct wound care/dressing change technique				

Exhibit 9–14 continued

Possible Points	Actual Points		Yes	No	N/A	Comments
15	_____	g. No undue color change at site				
15	_____	h. Temperature—no undue changes at site				
15	_____	i. Wound/decubiti—no undue swelling or induration				
15	_____	j. Wound—decreasing in size				
15	_____	k. Drainage—none or controlled Data Source for #1a-k: Nurse's notes				
15	_____	l. Wound or decubiti cultures are:				
8	_____	i. Negative or				
8	_____	ii. Being treated with antibiotics per sensitivity report Data Source: Lab results				
12	_____	m. Activity promotes wound healing, within restrictions Data Source: Nurse's notes				
_____	_____	n. Patient or caregiver verbalizes:				
10	_____	i. Complications				
10	_____	ii. Preventive measures Data Source: Nurse's notes				
		2. Does the record indicate that (unless physician orders are evident with specific parameters to the contrary):				
12	_____	a. Blood pressure is maintained between 90/60–160/90 mm Hg				
12	_____	b. Pulse is 60–90 beats per minute and regular				
12	_____	c. Respiratory rate is 12–24 breaths per minute at rest and unlabored				
14	_____	d. Temperature is 96.4–99°F orally Data Source: Nurse's notes				

continues

Exhibit 9–14 continued

Possible Points	*Actual Points*	
		Instructions to #2: If vital signs are outside of stated parameters, the auditor may still give points if the record indicates the nurse noted the change, recorded an explanation, and intervened with notification to the physician.

Total
Points: Thresholds:
275   80%

Source: Courtesy of Vickie Trevarthan, RN, and Wanda Kerns, RN.

Exhibit 9–15 Sample—Diagnosis-Related Audit for Cancer (General)

SCOPE OF CARE:

- Cancer (primary diagnosis)
- Patient has been receiving services for at least 60 days

SIGNIFICANT ASPECTS OF CARE:

1. Teaching process
2. Assessment process

CLINICAL INDICATORS:

1. Structure Indicators: Compliance with protocols outside the nurse's control
2. Process Indicators: Compliance with protocols within the nurse's control
3. Outcome Indicators: Result of indicators and patient compliance

Exhibit 9–15 continued

THRESHOLDS (evaluation of clinical indicators):

1. Structure Indicators: 85% compliance
2. Process Indicators: 98% compliance
3. Outcome Indicators: 80% compliance

INSTRUCTIONS:

- Check yes when criterion has been met.
- Check no when criterion was not met.
- Check N/A when the criterion does not apply to the patient or when the patient's primary diagnosis changes as a result of an acute episode or document noncompliance. Surveyors are instructed to reduce the points allocated to N/A questions for threshold compliance.

Possible Points	*Actual Points*		Yes	No	N/A	Comments
		PART I: Structure Indicators (66 points)				
5	_____	1. Does the record indicate that teaching was directed to the primary caregiver? Data Source: First seven visit notes				
10	_____	2. Are contents of home health aide (HHA) assignments individualized? Data Source: Last HHA assignment sheet				
9	_____	3. Were identified safety measures diagnosis related? Data Source: Plan of treatment/psychosocial factors				
8	_____	4. Is patient history reflective of primary diagnosis? Data Source: Nurse assessment (history)				
10	_____	5. Are the goals related to the primary diagnosis?				
4	_____	a. Are the stated goals measurable?				
4	_____	b. Are they stated with a time frame? Data Source: Plan of treatment				
6	_____	6. Is equipment identified? Data Source: Psychosocial factors of RN assessment				

continues

Exhibit 9–15 continued

Possible Points	Actual Points		Yes	No	N/A	Comments
10		7. Is care plan reflective of primary diagnosis?				

| Total Points: 66 | | Thresholds: 85% | |

Possible Points	Actual Points		Yes	No	N/A	Comments
		PART II: Process Indicators (155 points)				
		1. Does the record indicate patient or caregiver was taught:				
		a. Medications:				
5		i. Schedule (drug, dosage, route, and time)				
5		ii. Actions				
5		iii. Side effects				
		b. Diet/hydration:				
5		i. High protein, unless contraindicated				
5		ii. High carbohydrate, unless contra-indicated				
5		iii. High fluid, unless contraindicated				
5		iv. Supplemental feedings as indicated				
10		c. Activity to promote circulation, within limitation				
10		d. Bowel program, with constipation or diarrhea				
10		e. Bladder program, with incontinence				
9		f. Skin care, preventive measures				
7		g. Disease process or progression				
7		i. What to report?				
13		h. Emergency measures (if no do not resuscitate order)				

Exhibit 9–15 continued

Possible Points	Actual Points		Yes	No	N/A	Comments
11	_____	i. Signs and symptoms of other complications Data Source: First 60 days of service nurse's notes except emergency measures, which should be on first visit note				
15	_____	2. Were identified safety measures taught? Data Source: Nurse's notes first 7 visits				
8	_____	3. Was equipment used checked for safety? Data Source: Psychological factors				
20	_____	4. Was care plan updated with pertinent changes and with dates and initials?				

| Total Points
155 | _____ | Thresholds:
98%   _____ | | | | |

Possible Points	Actual Points		Yes	No	N/A	Comments
		PART III: Outcome Indicators (188 points) 1. Does the record indicate: a. Patient or caregiver verbalizes understanding of medication:				
4	_____	i. Schedule				
4	_____	ii. Actions				
4	_____	iii. Side effects				
4	_____	iv. Compliance				
15	_____	b. Patient or caregiver verbalizes understanding of disease process				
14	_____	c. i. Weight stable +/– 5 pounds, unless weight gain or loss desirable				

continues

Exhibit 9–15 continued

Possible Points	Actual Points		Yes	No	N/A	Comments
14	_____	ii. Patient or caregiver compliant with diet, fluids, and/or supplemental feedings				
15	_____	d. Pain none/controlled				
13	_____	e. No deterioration in skin integrity since admission				
13	_____	f. Activity within patient tolerance level				
13	_____	g. Bladder—continent and/or effective management				
13	_____	h. Bowel—without constipation/diarrhea and/or effective management				
11	_____	i. Patient or caregiver verbalizes understanding of other complications and relationship to disease process.				
		2. Does the record indicate that (unless physician orders are evident with specific parameters to the contrary):				
12	_____	a. Blood pressure is maintained between 90/60–160/90 mm Hg				
12	_____	b. Pulse is 60–90 beats per minute and regular				
12	_____	c. Respiratory rate is 12–24 breaths per minute at rest and unlabored				
15	_____	d. Temperature is 96.4–99°F orally				
		Data Source: Nurse's notes				

Instructions to #2: If vital
signs are outside of stated
parameters, the auditor may
still give points if the record

Exhibit 9–15 continued

Possible Points	*Actual Points*	
		indicates the nurse noted the change, recorded an explanation, and intervened with notification to the physician.
Total Points: 188 _____	_____	Thresholds: 80% _____ _____

Source: Courtesy of Vickie Trevarthan, RN, Stone Mountain, Georgia.

Exhibit 9–16 Sample—Diagnosis-Related Audit for Inflammatory Bowel Disease

SCOPE OF CARE:

- Inflammatory bowel disease (primary diagnosis)
- Patient has been receiving services for at least 30 days

SIGNIFICANT ASPECTS OF CARE:

1. Teaching process
2. Assessment process
3. Treatment protocol

CLINICAL INDICATORS:

1. Structure Indicators: Compliance with protocols outside the nurse's control
2. Process Indicators: Compliance with protocols within the nurse's control
3. Outcome Indicators: Result of indicators and patient compliance

THRESHOLDS (evaluation of clinical indicators):

1. Structure Indicators: 85% compliance
2. Process Indicators: 98% compliance
3. Outcome Indicators: 80% compliance

continues

Exhibit 9–16 continued

INSTRUCTIONS:

- Check yes when criterion has been met.
- Check no when criterion was not met.
- Check N/A when the criterion does not apply to the patient or when the patient's primary diagnosis changes as a result of an acute episode or document noncompliance. Surveyors are instructed to reduce the points allocated to N/A questions for threshold compliance.

Possible Points	Actual Points		Yes	No	N/A	Comments
		PART I: Structure Indicators (66 points)				
5		1. Does the record indicate that teaching was directed to the primary caregiver? Data Source: First seven visit notes				
10		2. Are contents of home health aide (HHA) assignments individualized? Data Source: Last HHA assignment sheet				
9		3. Were safety measures identified as indicative of diagnosis? Data Source: Plan of treatment/psychosocial factors				
8		4. Is patient history reflective of primary diagnosis? Data Source: Nurse assessment (history)				
10		5. Are the goals related to the primary diagnosis?				
4		a. Are the stated goals measurable?				
4		b. Are they stated with a time frame? Data Source: Plan of treatment				
6		6. Is equipment identified? Data Source: Psychosocial factors of RN assessment				
10		7. Is care plan reflective of primary diagnosis?				

Total
Points:
66 _____

Thresholds:
85% _____

Exhibit 9–16 continued

Possible Points	Actual Points		Yes	No	N/A	Comments
		PART II: Process Indicators (236 points)				
		1. Does the record indicate patient or caregiver was taught:				
		a. Medications:				
5	___	i. Schedule (drug, dosage, route, and time)				
5	___	ii. Actions				
5	___	iii. Side effects				
		b. Nutrition				
7	___	i. Balanced diet— Bland, high protein, low residue, unless otherwise indicated				
7	___	ii. High calorie— Unless otherwise indicated				
14	___	c. Fluid intake to prevent dehydration				
7	___	d. Signs/symptoms of dehydration				
		e. Parenteral fluids:				
15	___	i. Administration				
15	___	ii. Infection control precautions with administration				
12	___	f. Activity to meet levels of disability				
7	___	g. i. Signs/symptoms of exacerbation of disease				
7	___	ii. What to report to physician/nurse (bloody stools, diarrhea, constipation, abdominal distention)				
		h. Skin care:				
6	___	i. Per order				
6	___	ii. Preventive measures				
12	___	i. Signs/symptoms of electrolyte imbalance				
13	___	j. Stress factors				

continues

Exhibit 9–16 continued

Possible Points	Actual Points		Yes	No	N/A	Comments
13		k. Signs/symptoms of weakness/fatigue				
12		l. Information about disease process				
11		m. Other complications				
14		n. Emergency measures Data Source: First 30 days of service nurse's notes except emergency measures, which should be on first visit note				
15		2. Were identified safety measures taught? Data Source: Nurse's notes first seven visits				
8		3. Was equipment used checked for safety? Data Source: Psychosocial factors				
20		4. Was care plan updated with pertinent changes and with dates and initials?				

Total Points: 236 ___   Thresholds: 98% ___

Possible Points	Actual Points		Yes	No	N/A	Comments
		PART III: Outcome Indicators (300 points)				
		1. Patient or caregiver verbalizes understanding of medication:				
5		a. Schedule (drug, dosage, route, and time)				
5		b. Actions				
5		c. Side effects				
5		d. Compliance				
15		2. Patient or caregiver verbalizes understanding of dietary management				
15		3. Weight stable +/– 2 pounds, unless weight gain desirable				
15		4. Hydration maintained				

Exhibit 9–16 continued

Possible Points	Actual Points		Yes	No	N/A	Comments
13		5. Nausea/vomiting—none/controlled				
14		6. Patient or caregiver verbalizes understanding of teaching parenteral fluids administration				
14		7. Patient or caregiver demonstrates administration of parenteral fluid				
14		8. Patient or caregiver demonstrates infection control procedures with parenteral fluid administration				
12		9. Patient or caregiver demonstrates skin care per order				
12		10. Skin intact				
11		11. Patient or caregiver verbalizes preventive skin care measures				
14		12. Patient or caregiver verbalizes understanding of disease exacerbation				
14		13. Patient or caregiver verbalizes understanding of what to report to physician/nurse (bloody stool, diarrhea, constipation, and abdominal distention)				
13		14. Pain none/controlled				
		Data Source for #1–14: Nurse's notes				
7		15. Lab values:				
7		a. Electrolytes, within normal limits or within parameters set by physician for patient				
7		b. Complete blood count, within normal limits or within parameters set by physician for patient				
7		c. Biochemical profile 28, within normal limits or within parameters set by physician for patient				

continues

Exhibit 9–16 continued

Possible Points	Actual Points		Yes	No	N/A	Comments
		Data Source: Lab Results				
12	_____	16. Patient or caregiver verbalizes understanding of signs/symptoms of weakness/fatigue, allows time for sufficient rest periods				
13	_____	17. Patient or caregiver will be able to verbalize stress factors in life style				
		18. Does the record indicate that (unless physician orders are evident with specific parameters to the contrary):				
12	_____	a. Blood pressure is maintained between 90/60–160/90 mm Hg				
12	_____	b. Pulse is 60–90 beats per minute and regular				
12	_____	c. Respiratory rate is 12–24 breaths per minute and at rest and unlabored				
15	_____	d. Temperature is 96.4–99°F orally				
		Data Source for #16–18: Nurse's notes				

Instructions to #18: If vital signs are outside of stated parameters, the auditor may still give points if the record indicates the nurse noted the change, recorded an explanation, and intervened with notification to the physician.

Total Points: 300 _____

Thresholds: 80% _____

Source: Courtesy of Vickie Trevarthan, RN, and Wanda Kerns, RN.

Chapter 10

Utilization Review Audits

INTRODUCTION

Utilization review (UR) audits are perhaps the most necessary of all audit types because these functions and activities ensure payment. As mentioned earlier in this book, utilization review is a process by which appropriate utilization of services is validated in accordance with guidelines established by the payer source, including the efficient use of resources. "UR changes with the wind," is a statement often heard among quality assurance professionals. The impetus behind the many changes is government regulators and payer changes such as Health Maintenance Organizations (HMOs), Preferred Provider Organizations (PPOs), etc. Therefore, the issue of definition should be flexible. For purposes of this book and generally in the home care setting, UR is meant to be a review function covering the appropriateness of care in relation to the payer source.

As previously discussed, UR audits call for judgments; consequently, it is recommended that one nurse be responsible consistently for this functional area. Exhibit 10–1 is an example of the UR audit form for Medicare. Remember, this audit has a limited scope and should address only issues relative to qualifying criteria and other rules imposed by payers. Therefore, it is strongly recommended that the UR nurse have access to only those records that will accompany the Uniform Bill–82 (UB–82) or other invoices as prescribed by the payer.

If the UR nurse questions coverage issues with the limited documentation available, it is highly likely that the intermediary will request additional information. If the UR nurse has access to the entire medical record, the tendency will be to find the information being sought. The intermediary does not have access to the entire medical record in order to make a claims decision. Therefore, the UR nurse should not, for it will no doubt cloud the nurse's judgment regarding the appropriateness of documentation to be sent to the payer.

It is also recommended that the UR nurse review claims with supporting documentation attached before they are mailed to the fiscal intermediary using

Exhibit 10–1 Retrospective, Concurrent, and Prospective Utilization Review—Medicare

Page _____ of _____
Date of Review: _____
Branch: _____
weak: _____
acceptable: _____
unacceptable documentation: _____

Patient's Name	Nurse Responsible	Plan of Treatment and Voice Order Signed by Physician	Timely Home Health Aide Skilled Visit	Homebound Evident	Disciplines Reflective of Diagnosis and on Plans of Treatment	Record Reflective of Skilled Services Provided	Condition Justifying Utilization	Physician Validation of Practices Above/Below/Norm	Physician Appt.	Case Conference	Comments

Signature _____ Date

a random selection. The UR nurse is then in the same position as the intermediary and can make a judgment accordingly. This process is also a wonderful opportunity to teach and reinforce to staff the importance of appropriate documentation. This is an excellent opportunity to use the p chart for proportion defective.

The following are examples of specific UR questions by payer source. It is important to note that these questions will vary depending on the payer's focus.

MEDICARE*

1. Plan of Treatment (HCFA 485/486/487) and Verbal Orders—All physician orders must be dated and signed and incorporated into the medical record. All fields on the HCFA–485 series must be completed accurately in accordance with the patient's status and medical condition.
2. Timely Supervision of Home Health Aides (HHAs)—Supervisory visits for HHAs should be documented by the nurse, speech therapist, or physical therapist at least every 14 days. The notation should indicate whether the HHA is following the assigned tasks and whether the patient is meeting the goals established. It is also advisable to note whether the patient or family is satisfied with the HHA and the services being rendered.
3. Homebound Status—The Medicare records submitted to the fiscal intermediary must clearly indicate that the client has a physical or functional limitation that renders him or her unable to leave the home without the assistance of another person or an assistive device. The latest mandate from the Health Care Financing Administration (HCFA) will also allow patients to qualify for homebound status when the condition is such that it becomes unsafe for the patient to leave home. Consideration must also be given to the frequency and purpose that a client is leaving home.
4. Disciplines Ordered Reflective of Diagnosis—The HCFA–485 or HCFA–486 should be reviewed to ensure that all disciplines have been ordered that are medically indicated for the client's diagnosis and treatment. Review also should indicate when disciplines ordered are not medically indicated and necessary. If this is the case, a denial could result from the intermediary.
5. Record Reflective of Skilled Services Provided—The documentation provided should reflect that skilled services were provided and are in accordance with physician orders. The UR nurse should pay close attention to the HCFA–487 for updated information.

---

*Note that the following information on Medicare is subject to change as regulations are revised.

6. Condition Justifying Utilization—The plan of treatment should document that the services ordered and rendered are medically indicated and necessary for the client's diagnosis and condition according to guidelines issued by HCFA.
7. Physician Validation of Practices Above or Below the Norm—If services ordered and rendered are above or below normal (as set by the American Medical Association) for the diagnoses and condition of the client, a validation letter from the physician should be included in the record. For example, due to large amounts of sediment, a physician may want a Foley catheter changed every two weeks.
8. Comments—The UR nurse should use a comments section to indicate why a deficiency was given. It is also used when care is becoming routine or nonskilled and when discharge or transfer of patient should be considered.

THIRD-PARTY PAYERS

Private insurance companies and other third-party payers are putting more restrictions on coverage than ever before. Many of the major carriers follow Medicare guidelines very closely. This effort to curb cost by limiting utilization places the UR nurse in an expanding role. The UR nurse must not only assure the agency of payment by conforming to the payer's guidelines, but must also become the client's advocate.

Client advocacy will most often be reflected when the UR nurse attempts to get the insurance company to cover additional services. UR nurses should be aggressive in their attempts to gain coverage for the agency's clients.

Exhibit 10–2 is an example of a UR form for third-party payers.

1. Plan of Treatment—The plan of treatment (POT) should be complete and include all orders for services and treatments being rendered. Homebound status is not always required but assists to support the need for home care. The POT and verbal orders must be signed prior to submitting to the payer.
2. Discipline Reflective of Diagnosis—The POT should be reviewed to ensure that all disciplines have been ordered that are medically indicated for the patient's diagnosis and treatment. Review also should indicate when disciplines ordered are not medically indicated and necessary.
3. Record Reflective of Skilled Services Provided—The record should document that the services provided are skilled and in accordance with physician orders.
4. Condition Justifying Utilization—The POT should document that the services ordered and rendered are medically indicated for the patient's

Exhibit 10–2 Retrospective, Concurrent, and Prospective Utilization Review—Private Insurance

Y = Yes
N = No
NA = Nonapplicable
POT = Plan of Treatment
VO = Voice Order

Page _____ of _____
Date of Review: _____
Branch: _____
weak: _____
acceptable: _____
unacceptable documentation: _____

Patient's Name	Case Mgr. Init.	POT & VO signed by physician	POT complete	Disciplines reflective of diagnosis	Record reflects need for continued care/services	Record reflective of services ordered	Condition justifying utilization	Physician validation medical necessity	Comments

Signature _____ Date _____

diagnosis and condition. The record also should document that care ordered and provided can only be rendered by a licensed nurse.

5. Physician Validation of Practices Above or Below the Norm—If services ordered and rendered are above or below the normal for the diagnoses and condition of the patient, a validation letter from the physician should be included in the record. The physician may also validate that without skilled services in the home, hospitalization could be the alternative.

6. Comments—This section is used to indicate why a deficiency has been given. It is also used to document when care is becoming nonskilled or when discharge or transfer of patient is indicated.

PATIENT ADVOCACY

The UR program is gaining increasing attention as an ethical issue for two reasons:

1. limitations on access to health care
2. efforts to reduce cost

Increasing numbers of individuals lack health care insurance, which limits their access to the delivery system. Inpatient stays have dramatically changed since prospective payment and managed care initiatives. Hospital care has become aggressive in order to stabilize patients rapidly so they can be cared for in a less expensive setting. The result has been that patients, primarily the elderly, have been discharged sooner and sicker than ever before. The rapid growth of home care can be attributed, at least in part, to this environmental change. The UR nurse's role in patient advocacy will continue to increase as the health care dollar is tightened even further.

This advocacy role cannot be overemphasized. It would appear that some managed care payers are more concerned with cost containment than with the condition of a patient whom they generally have never seen. The UR nurse has the responsibility to refuse to admit a patient if, after assessment, it is determined that the patient requires more care than the payer is willing to approve. This is a critical issue and one on which a great deal of discussion should take place.

Ethically, once the agency accepts a patient and begins to render care, it is obligated to continue that care unless other appropriate arrangements can be made for the care and treatment of the individual. If there is no insurance coverage and the client is unable to pay, it will be extremely difficult to find another provider to continue the treatment.

For this reason, the UR nurse must be adept at negotiating with payers and not be intimidated by threats of sending the patient elsewhere. If the agency cannot render adequate medical care within the limitations set by the payer, the client should be refused on those grounds.

OTHER ROLES OF THE UR NURSE

In addition to audit process and patient advocacy roles, the UR nurse also should play a key role in staff development. The UR nurse knows which nurses are having problems with what issues. The comments written by the UR nurse on audit forms should be acted upon immediately to save the agency from unnecessary reimbursement denials. The nurses responsible for deficiencies should use the information as a learning opportunity. The staff development department should be given a synopsis of findings to review in inservice programming.

A final recommendation is that the UR nurse be made responsible for all communication from and to the medical review departments of the intermediary or insurance companies. This action will heighten the agency's ability to speak with a consistent voice and will centralize the knowledge gained into the most appropriate person. This is not to say, however, that knowledge gained should not be shared. On the contrary, all knowledge gained by the UR nurse should be disseminated to the staff as expeditiously as possible through the staff development process.

The utilization review nurse becomes the agency's standard bearer. This nurse is highly specialized and should, above all else, seek to teach the staff appropriate documentation skills. This nurse, who advocates the client's right to have medically necessary services rendered in the home setting, will become one of the most valued employees on staff.

TRENDS IN UTILIZATION REVIEW

Hospitals have long had severity of illness or acuity systems. This level of professionalism has not yet been achieved in the home care industry. The industry has the capability of developing such a system using the data base that HCFA has accumulated from certified agencies. No doubt this data base will be utilized in the eventual development of a prospective payment plan for home care.

LEGAL CONSIDERATIONS

Concurrent UR is a valuable tool of risk management. Potential problems can be corrected while the patient is still in treatment and before litigation is necessary. The UR nurse should be reporting any trends identified to the quality assurance (QA) and risk management departments. As mentioned in the discussion on the patient advocacy role, the UR nurse should be the final decision maker regarding the acceptance of a patient for continuing treatment. This decision should not be made by a nonclinical person.

Chapter 11

Field Review Audits

PROCESS AUDITS

The process of clinical surveillance is intended to validate the competence of the nurse or other staff in areas of technical expertise, ability to teach, and compliance with policies and procedures relating to patient care. Trends from these audits identify process problems where opportunities for improvement exist. Process audits make an exceptionally good tool for quantifying the evaluation process for promotion purposes.

The first process audit examined here is a field audit of a nurse. The format should follow closely those of the quality assurance audits, in that the scope should be defined as well as significant aspects and indicators. Exhibit 11–1 provides an example of this type of field audit.

Since a field review audit is conducted as an observation, the infection control process must be done while the nurse is conducting the home visit. As a prerequisite, the supervisor or person conducting the review should have the client's consent before performing this audit. The nurse rendering care should obtain such consent prior to the review process.

The purpose of Part I of this audit is to validate compliance with standards imposed by the agency regarding infection control, for example. (See Exhibit 11–2.) Additionally, the agency should validate the nurse's ability to appropriately teach medications. Before the reviewer goes into the home with the nurse, the medical record should be reviewed to gain a complete understanding of the patient's medical condition and knowledge, according to the record, of the medications the patient is currently taking. With this done, the audit may proceed.

Part II of this audit is outcome oriented, although process is being tested. (See Exhibit 11–3.) Validation of a nurse's teaching ability can be tested only by finding out the patient's level of knowledge.

Each of the questions in Exhibit 11–3 provides for a discussion that is designed to elicit an appropriate response. Instructions are also provided where indicated.

Exhibit 11–1 Field Audit Format

SCOPE:

Patients who have:

1. High frequency (3x/week or more registered nurse [RN]) admission within 30 days of audit
2. Long-term, low frequency (1x/month or less) admission 3 months or more
3. Multidiscipline (RN and home health aide [HHA] at least) admission within 60 days (preferably clients with therapies)

SIGNIFICANT ASPECTS OF CARE:

1. Infection control process
2. Teaching medications
3. Technical procedure

INDICATORS:

1. Structure Indicators: Nurse follows protocol for home visit and mutually agreeable appointment times
2. Process Indicators:
   a. Infection control—bag technique, cleaning equipment (if present), handwashing
   b. Verification of correct medication regimen
   c. Teaching per care plan
   d. Observation of specific procedure
3. Outcome Indicators:
   a. Patient understanding of treatment plan and goals
   b. Patient knowledge of medication regimen
   c. Patient knowledge of safety factors and emergency protocol
   d. Patient perception of staff compliance with visit appointments

THRESHOLDS:

Structure Indicators: 95% compliance
Process Indicators: 98% compliance
Outcomes Indicators: 90% compliance

Part III of the field audit is designed to be able to validate any procedure. (See Exhibit 11–4.) This tool is generic but should not be point scored as Parts I and II. It is impossible to have a specific technical procedure audit tool for each of the thousands of procedures that may be done in the home. Therefore, a generic tool, while it will highlight problem areas, is not objective, and the outcome will largely depend on the competence level of the person conducting the review.

Exhibit 11–2 Generic Field Audit—Part I

Possible Points	Actual Points		Yes	No	N/A	Comments
		Process Observations: Generic (30 points)				
		1. Infection Control				
4	___	a. Was the nurse observed using proper handwashing technique?				
4	___	b. Was the nurse observed using proper bag technique?				
4	___	c. Was the nurse observed using proper infection control on thermometer?				
4	___	d. Was the nurse observed using proper infection control on stethoscope?				
4	___	e. Was the nurse observed using proper infection control on sphygmomanometer?				
10	___	2. Are the medications the patient is currently taking the same as indicated in the medical record? (Instructions: Do not count any medication changes since last visit)				

Source: Courtesy of Vickie Trevarthan, RN, Stone Mountain, Georgia.

For those procedures that an agency performs frequently, it is recommended that a specific audit tool be developed utilizing the *Lippincott Manual of Nursing Practice,* most recently revised edition. This type of audit does not lend itself to the format of quality assurance audits, since the scope is already defined by virtue of the procedure. Additionally, the entire audit is a process audit in a step-by-step procedure.

These audits should have the highest thresholds since it is assumed that most nurses are competent in performing basic nursing procedures. The exception would be a procedure never done by the nurse previously or done years before. In these cases, this audit is a systematic method the agency can use to validate the nurse's technical skill on a procedure or as a teaching guide.

When using specific procedures in step-by-step format, point scoring is essential to calculate the threshold. (See Exhibit 11–5.)

Exhibit 11–3 Generic Field Audit—Part II

Possible Points	Actual Points		Yes	No	N/A	Comments
		Outcome: Patient Interview (70 points)				
5	_____	1. Does the patient know the treatment plan? Discussion: What is the nurse doing?				
5	_____	2. Does the patient know the goals of care? Discussion: Why is the nurse doing it?				
10	_____	3. Does the patient know his or her role in treatment in absence of nurse? Discussion: What are you supposed to do when the nurse isn't here?				
		(Instructions: For questions 4–7, any means the patient has of identifying medication is acceptable, but he or she must be able to identify each treatment)				
10	_____	4. Does the patient or caregiver know what medications to take? Discussion: What medicine are you taking? _____				
10	_____	5. Does the patient or caregiver know when and how much of each medication to take? Discussion: When do you take each medicine, and how much of each do you take? _____				
5	_____	6. Does the patient or caregiver know why he or she is taking each medication? Discussion: Why are you taking each of these pills? _____				
5	_____	7. Does the patient or caregiver know side effects of each medication?				

Exhibit 11–3 continued

Possible Points	*Actual Points*		Yes	No	N/A	Comments
		Discussion: Do you know what the side effects of your medication are? _____				
10	___	8. Does the patient or caregiver understand emergency procedure? Discussion: If something bad happens or you get very sick, what would you do? _____				
5	___	9. Does the patient or caregiver know safety precautions? (Instructions: If safety hazard observed in home, specifically use that as an example) Discussion: What has the nurse asked you to change in your surroundings to prevent accidents?				
5	___	10. Does staff schedule in advance convenient visit times?				

Exhibit 11–4 Generic Field Audit—Part III
(Process Indicators: Nursing Standards of Care, Procedure Specific)

Instruction: Where specific procedure audit tool is unavailable, use commentary for deficiencies.

_____   _____
           Nurse   Surveyor

Specific procedure _____ Date _____

Was the procedure followed in accordance with standard of nursing practice?
YES____ NO____
If no, list specific deficiency:

_____
_____
_____
_____
_____
_____
_____

It cannot be emphasized enough that this type of technical procedure audit should be utilized to validate a new skill for a nurse. In this dynamic age of new technologies in the home, it is the provider's responsibility to ensure the competence of those rendering care.

In accordance with the Deming model, the design and redesign of new services should always include the review process. For example, if the agency were going to begin blood transfusions in the home, the nurses who would be responsible should be validated as having technical competence before the service is offered to the general public. This step not only ensures quality, but reduces the agency's risk of potential liability.

Exhibit 11–5 Skilled Nurse Technical Home Audit—Catheterizations
(Female Indwelling Urinary Catheter)

Branch _____   Date _____
Nurse _____   Surveyor _____

	Possible Points	Actual Points
1. Check that catheter size is in accordance with physician order.	5	
2. Put on nonsterile gloves.	3	
3. Observe genital area for rashes or lesions, odor, color (e.g., redness, bruises), drainage, and local edema.	3	
4. Cleanse external urethral meatus and surrounding area with soap and water.	3	
5. Remove gloves and discard.	3	
6. Wash hands.	3	
7. Remove disposable tray from plastic bag.	3	
8. Open catheter tray using aseptic technique.	3	
9. Carefully remove underpad and place under patient with absorbent side up.	3	
10. Pull back one side of the catheter package using aseptic technique.	3	
11. Put on sterile gloves.	5	
12. Using syringe found in top of catheter tray, check catheter balloon for inflatability by instilling 10 mL of distilled water into plastic balloon valve; then withdraw solution.	3	
13. Pour iodophor or packaged solution over rayon balls. Squeeze lubricant into tray.	3	
14. Drape patient with fenestrated drape.	3	
15. With one hand, hold the labia back from the meatus.	5	

Exhibit 11–5 continued

	Possible Points	*Actual Points*
16. Using other hand, take forceps and pick up absorbent rayon balls. Cleansing strokes should be made from front to back of the perineum, using each swab for one stroke only. Clean the center of the area first, then the sides.	5	
17a. With uncontaminated hand, take catheter from package, lubricate tip, and insert gently into meatus in an upward and backward direction.	5	
17b. If urethra is not entered correctly the first time, the catheter should be discarded and a new one obtained for next attempt.	5	
18. Insert approximately one inch further after urine begins to flow.	5	
19. Instill appropriate or ordered amount of distilled water into plastic balloon.	3	
20. Assess urine for amount, color, character, odor, and hematuria.	5	
21. Allow urine to flow until a maximum of 500 mL has been withdrawn (skip #21 and #22 if less than 500 mL of urine is obtained).	3	
22. Clamp catheter.	3	
23. Withdraw remaining urine at a volume of 200mL/ 30 minutes.	3	
24. Save specimen for lab examination, if ordered.	3	
25. Tape catheter to drainage tube at catheter/ drainage tube connection using 1" tape. Apply tape length-wise rather than wrapping to prevent disconnecting from catheter.	2	
26. Remove gloves and discard with used materials.	2	
27. Using tape as label, apply to catheter the name of the person performing procedure and the date.	2	
28. Wash hands.	3	

Final Score _____
Possible Score _____
Threshold _____

Threshold: 98%

Source: Courtesy of Vickie Trevarthan, RN, Stone Mountain, Georgia.

Chapter 12

Infection Prevention and Control

Prevention and control of infection in the home setting is a challenge for health care personnel and families. Patients are at risk of acquiring infections at home as well as in the hospital, even though pathogens are generally less numerous and less severe in the home environment. Chronic or debilitating disease, age, altered defense mechanisms, therapeutic modalities, and medical devices and procedures all predispose patients to infection. Patients must be protected from the occurrence or spread of infection, and families and friends must be protected from individuals with an infectious process. Everyone is responsible for the prevention and control of infection.

Iganz Semmelweis demonstrated in the 1840s the effectiveness of handwashing with an aseptic solution. Today, despite modern technology and scientific advances, handwashing is still the most significant combatant against the spread of disease.

The Centers for Disease Control and Prevention (CDCP) published the first set of definitions for nosocomial infections in 1969 and shortly thereafter recommended that all hospitals practice surveillance techniques for the control and prevention of infection. The CDCP, as the leading authority on infection prevention and control, came under strong criticism in the early 1980s when some large hospitals were having difficulty in establishing an adequate number of infection control nurses (e.g., one full-time equivalent for every 250 beds).

The critics were silenced, however, when the CDCP's *Study of the Efficacy of Nosocomial Infection Control* (SENIC) strongly substantiated the necessity of surveillance to reduce infection rates. The conclusion was that without an organized and routine surveillance system, even the most vigorously controlled policies and procedures are unlikely to be successful.

While the SENIC project was a study involving hospitals only, its principles and concepts are applicable to home care. For this reason, let us begin with a fundamental review of universal precautions.

UNIVERSAL PRECAUTIONS

Universal infection control precautions are designed to prevent and control the spread of disease-causing microorganisms among patients, caregivers, and other persons. Since agent and host factors are more difficult to control, interruption of the chain of infection is directed primarily at the mode of transmission through the use of barrier protection. The transmission of disease, defined as any mechanism by which an infectious agent is spread through the environment or to another person, requires three elements:

1. a source of infecting organism
2. a susceptible host (client)
3. a means of transmission for the organism

The source of an infecting agent may be the family, health care personnel, or visitors, and may include persons with acute disease, persons in the incubation period of a disease, or persons who are colonized by an infectious agent with no apparent disease. Other sources of infection can be the client's own microbial flora, and contaminated inanimate objects in the environment such as equipment and medications.

A client's resistance to pathogenic microorganisms varies greatly. Some may be immune or able to resist colonization by an infectious agent, while others exposed to the same agent may become asymptomatic carriers or develop the clinical disease. Those clients treated with certain antibiotics, steroids, radiation, or immunosuppressive agents may be particularly prone to infection. Age, chronic disease, acute disease, traumatic injury, or surgical procedures can also make a person more susceptible.

Microorganisms are transmitted by various routes, and the same one may be transmitted by more than one route. Current infection control precautions have been designed to reduce physical and emotional isolation as much as possible, as well as to protect health care workers and others from transmissible disease.

Everyone is responsible for using recommended precautions, including patients who have the responsibility for compliance. Appropriate measures should be explained to the client, family, and caregivers. One important general responsibility is handwashing. Infractions by some are sufficient to negate the conscientious efforts of others. The maxim "The chain is no stronger than the weakest link" holds true.

The next sections look at the various components of infection control and precaution techniques in general terms. For specific precautions by disease state, consult the CDCP.

HANDWASHING

Handwashing is to be done on entering and leaving the client's home and additionally as needed. Hands should be lathered with friction for at least ten seconds. As discussed earlier, this is one of the most important measures of control and prevention of infections.

Examples of times when handwashing is indicated follow:

- before and after touching wounds
- after situations during which microbial contamination of hands is likely to occur, especially those involving contact with mucous membranes, blood or body fluids, secretions, or excretions
- after touching inanimate sources that are likely to be contaminated with virulent or epidemiologically important microorganisms (these sources include urine-measuring devices or secretion-collection apparatuses)
- after taking care of an infected patient or one who is likely to be colonized with microorganisms of special clinical or epidemiologic significance, for example, multiresistant bacteria

Employees should have a dispenser of liquid soap for use. The dispenser should be cleaned and filled with fresh soap when empty.

Hands are to be dried with a disposable towel. The water faucet is to be turned off with the paper towel. These supplies should be issued to every caregiver of the agency as needed.

BAG TECHNIQUE

The nursing bag should be used in accordance with the following directions:

1. The contents of the nursing bag should be held to an absolute minimum, reflecting only those items needed routinely for patient care.
2. The inside pouch of the bag must be kept aseptic at all times and should not be entered until hands are thoroughly cleaned.
3. The outside pouches can be used for any reusable items and disposal items as deemed necessary by the nurse.
4. The inside of the bag must be thoroughly cleansed with alcohol at least once a month and additionally as necessary. The outside may be cleaned with soap and water.
5. The bag is never placed on the floor under any circumstances.
6. Upon entering the client's home, place the bag on a *hard* surface covered with newspaper.

7. Remove coat; fold it with the outside exposed; and place it on a hard surface away from the bag area.
8. Designate a "clean" and "dirty" area on the paper near the bag.
9. Remove soap and towels from the side pocket, and wash hands thoroughly using proper handwashing techniques.
10. Open aseptic center pouch, and remove all items needed for the visit. Place these items on "clean" side of the newspaper, and close the bag.
11. Use paper towels as protective shields while in the performance of various patient care functions.
12. Dispose of all "dirty" items properly.
13. After care is given, clean all equipment thoroughly with alcohol.
14. Clean hands again using proper technique, and return clean items to bag.
15. The bag should be kept locked in the trunk while not in use.

PROTECTIVE PRECAUTIONS

All staff must wear gloves when coming in contact with any body fluids or secretions; that is feces, sputum, saliva, blood, urine, wound drainage, etc.

Employees should protect their uniforms from contamination by using disposable aprons as appropriate. Soiled, dirty linen is not to come in contact with the employee's uniform. Employees will not sit on the floor at any time during the client's care unless the floor is covered with a paper or clean linen and the client cannot be cared for from another position.

ENGINEERING CONTROLS

Whenever possible, engineering controls should be used as the primary method to reduce caregiver exposure to harmful substances. The preferred approach in engineering controls is to use to the fullest extent feasible intrinsically safe substances, procedures, or devices—for example, the sharps needle disposal. Using disposable, puncture-resistant containers for used needles, blades, etc., is an alternative engineering control technique. This technique isolates cut and needlestick injury hazards from the caregiver.

SHARP INSTRUMENTS AND DISPOSABLE ITEMS

The following precautions should be observed with sharps:

1. Needles should not be recapped, purposely bent or broken by hand, removed from disposable syringes, or otherwise manipulated by hand.

2. After they are used, disposable syringes and needles, scalpel blades, and other sharp items should be placed in puncture-resistant containers for disposal.
3. Puncture-resistant containers should be provided for all personnel needing them, and personnel are to have sharp disposals available in order to dispose of all sharps immediately following use.
4. Sharp disposals shall be constructed so that they will not spill their contents if knocked over and will not themselves allow injuries when handled.

STERILE DISPOSABLE SUPPLIES

Sterile disposable supplies should be used, eliminating the need for any sterilization. Items that touch only intact skin (e.g., blood pressure cuffs and other medical accessories) rarely, if ever, transmit disease. Cleaning of these items should be done with alcohol after care is given.

PRECAUTIONS WITH LABORATORY SPECIMENS

Blood and other body fluids from *all* patients should be considered infective. To supplement the universal blood and body fluid precautions the following precautions are recommended for health care workers when collecting laboratory specimens:

1. All specimens of blood and body fluid should be put in a well-constructed container with a secure lid to prevent leaking during transport. Care should be taken when collecting each specimen to avoid contaminating the outside of the container or the laboratory form accompanying the specimen.
2. Use of needles and syringes should be limited to situations in which there is no alternative, and the recommendations for preventing injuries are outlined under sharp instruments.

Implementation of universal blood and body fluid precautions for all clients eliminates the need for warning labels on specimens since blood and other body fluids from all clients should be considered infective.

PERSONAL PROTECTIVE EQUIPMENT

Personal protective clothing and equipment need to be tailored to provide protection for specific tasks. Impervious gowns, gloves, eyewear, face shields, masks, and mouthpieces for CPR should be made available and issued as required equipment for every employee in contact with clients.

1. Gloves—The use of disposable gloves is indicated for procedures where body fluids are handled in the following circumstances:
   - if the health care worker has cuts, abraded skin, chapped hands, dermatitis, or the like
   - when examining abraded or nonintact skin or clients with active bleeding
   - during invasive procedures
   - during all cleaning of body fluids and decontaminating procedures
   - note the following:
     — Gloves must be of appropriate material, usually intact latex or intact vinyl, of appropriate quality for the procedures performed, and of appropriate size for each health care worker.
     — Employers shall not wash or disinfect sterile or examination gloves for reuse.
     — No gloves shall be used if they are peeling, cracked, or discolored, or if they have punctures, tears, or other evidence of deterioration.
2. Gowns—The use of gowns, aprons, or lab coats is required when splashes to skin or clothing with body fluids are likely to occur. Gowns (including surgical gowns) shall be made of or lined with impervious material and shall protect all areas of exposed skin.
3. Masks and Eye Protectors—The use of masks and protective eyewear or face shields is required when contamination of mucosal membranes (eyes, mouth, or nose) with body fluids such as splashes or aerosolization of such material (e.g., vigorous wound irrigations or nebulizer treatments) is likely to occur. They are not required for routine care.
4. Resuscitation Equipment—Mouthpieces, pocket masks, resuscitation bags, or other ventilation devices should be provided for all field staff where the need for resuscitation is possible. This will minimize the need for emergency mouth-to-mouth resuscitation.

The personal protective equipment described should be used when performing invasive procedures to avoid exposure. When a health care worker's skin or mucous membranes may come in contact with body fluids, gowns, masks, and eye protection should be worn.

INFECTIOUS WASTE

Infectious waste is defined as waste capable of producing an infectious disease. This definition requires a consideration of certain factors necessary for induction of disease. These factors include:

1. presence of a pathogen of sufficient virulence
2. dose
3. portal of entry
4. resistance of host

Therefore, for a waste to be infectious, it must contain pathogens with sufficient virulence and quantity so that exposure to the waste by a susceptible host could result in an infectious disease.

Identifying wastes for which special precautions are indicated is largely a matter of judgment about the relative risk of disease transmission. The most practical approach to the management of infectious waste is to identify those wastes with the potential for causing infection during their handling and disposal and for which some special precautions appear prudent, such as blood specimens or blood products.

Bulk blood, suctioned fluids, excretions, and secretions may be carefully poured down a drain connected to a sanitary sewer. Sanitary sewers may also be used to dispose of other infectious wastes capable of being ground and flushed into the sewer.

Infectious waste, in general, should either be incinerated or be autoclaved before disposal in a sanitary landfill.

Legislation does not yet exist that strictly prohibits the placing of untreated infectious waste in approved landfills. However, this type of disposal is discouraged strongly, especially for sharp-pointed items or "sharps." Consult the Environmental Protection Agency (EPA) guide for infectious waste management for specific disposal requirements. Waste management regulations in health care settings may also be obtained from state or local county health departments.

The following items are considered infectious waste that are likely to be encountered in home health care:

1. items with sharp points, commonly referred to as "sharps" (e.g., needles, syringes, scalpels, lancets)
2. blood and blood products
3. decubitus wound dressings and debridement materials

In general, the following sections may provide some guidance in the disposal of infectious waste.

Segregation of Infectious Waste

- Segregate infectious waste at the point of origin.
  1. Infectious waste should be separated from the general waste stream to ensure that these wastes will receive appropriate handling and treatment.

2. Infectious waste should be segregated from the general waste stream at the point of generation (i.e., the point at which the material becomes a waste).

- Provisions should be made for infectious waste with multiple hazards. These wastes should be segregated from the general infectious waste stream when additional or alternative treatment is required.
- Infectious waste should be discarded directly into containers or plastic bags that are clearly identifiable and distinguishable from the general waste stream.
    1. Containers should be marked with the universal biological hazard symbol (see below).
    2. Plastic bags also should be distinctively colored and/or marked with the universal biological hazard symbol.
    3. Red or orange colored plastic bags generally are used to identify infectious waste.

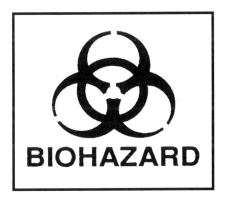

Packaging of Infectious Waste

- Infectious waste should be packaged in order to protect waste handlers and the public from possible injury and disease that may result from exposure to the waste.
    1. Infectious waste should be contained from the point of origin up to the point at which it is no longer infectious.
    2. The integrity of the packaging must be preserved through handling, storage, transportation, and treatment.
    3. Packaging should be appropriate for the type of waste to provide adequate waste containment.
- All discarded sharps (e.g., hypodermic needles, syringes, Pasteur pipettes, broken glass, scalpel blades) that have come into contact with infectious

agents during use in patient care present the double hazard of inflicting injury and inducing disease.

1. Sharps should be placed directly into impervious, rigid, leak-proof, and puncture-resistant containers to eliminate the hazard of physical injury.
2. Clipping of needles is *not* recommended.
3. Suitable container materials for sharps are glass, metal, rigid plastic, wood, and heavy cardboard; containers should be compatible with selected treatment processes. Containers for sharps should be marked with the universal biohazard symbol and sealed before handling. Sharp containers should be incinerated following use.

- Use plastic bags that are impervious, tear-resistant, and distinctive in color or markings.
  1. Thickness and durability are two criteria frequently used to judge suitability of a plastic bag.
  2. Close and seal the top of each bag by taping or tying as appropriate for treatment or transport.
- Do not compact infectious waste or packaged infectious waste before treatment.
- Where an adequate sewer line is not available, place liquid wastes in capped or tightly sealed containers or flasks until local health officials can determine risk, if any, from dumping into septic tanks or other waste disposal systems.

Storage of Infectious Waste

1. Minimize storage time.
2. Use proper packaging that ensures containment of infectious waste and the exclusion of rodents and vermin.
3. Limit access to storage area to persons delivering trash or treating trash.
4. Post the universal biological hazard symbol on storage area door, waste containers, freezers, or refrigerators.

Transport of Infectious Waste

1. Avoid mechanical loading devices that may rupture packaged wastes.
2. Disinfect carts used to transfer wastes within the home setting (or agency) frequently with a 1:10 solution of bleach or any reputable germicidal cleaner. Adequate physical cleaning (i.e., elbow grease) is necessary for any disinfecting agent to work effectively.

3. Place all infectious waste into rigid or semirigid containers before transport off-site.
4. Transport infectious waste in closed leak-proof vehicles or dumpsters. Be sure to limit access to dumpster before pickup.

Disposal of Infectious Waste

Blood and other body fluids may be poured down the toilet in a home known to be connected to a functioning public sewer line where municipal secondary treatment is available. An individual toilet for a client is not required, but is recommended if the person has diarrhea. Disinfection of these liquid wastes before flushing can be accomplished by merely adding a bleach solution of approximately a 1:10 dilution. (Such disinfection is not required.)

Where an adequate sewer line is not available:

1. Place liquid wastes in capped or tightly sealed containers or flasks until local health officials can determine risk, if any, from dumping into septic tanks or other waste disposal systems.
2. Solvents and strong chemicals (including large quantities of disinfectants) should not be added to an on-site sewage management system in order to avoid destroying beneficial organisms necessary for digestion of waste.

CONTAMINATED EQUIPMENT

Any discarded equipment or parts that may be contaminated with infectious agents are considered contaminated equipment. These wastes include equipment used in client care. Contaminated equipment should be treated by steam sterilization, incineration, or chemical disinfection on-site (e.g., bleach soak or scrub down).

EMPLOYEE EXPOSURE

An important aspect of the infection control problem is the issue of employee exposure. Home health care employees can become infected through exposure to infected patients if proper precautions are not used. Home care employees could then transmit the infection to other susceptible clients, coworkers, family members, or other community contacts.

The primary concerns of the infection control program are:

1. preventing transmission of infection both to and from personnel and patients

2. preventing transmission of infection primarily from infected patients to
   personnel

Employee Exposure Category I

Category I employees perform tasks that involve exposure to blood, body
fluids, or tissues. All procedures or other job-related tasks that involve an
inherent potential for mucous membrane or skin contact with blood, body fluids,
or tissues, or a potential for spills or splashes of them, are Category I tasks. Use
of appropriate protective measures should be required for every employee
engaged in Category I tasks.

Category I employees include:

- skilled nurses (registered nurses and licensed practical nurses)
- home health aides
- certified nursing assistants

Employee Exposure Category II

Category II employees perform tasks that involve no exposure to blood, body
fluids, or tissues, but their employment may require performing unplanned
category I tasks. The normal work routine involves no exposure to blood, body
fluids, or tissues, but exposure or potential exposure may be required as a
condition of employment. Appropriate protective measures should be readily
available to every employee engaged in Category II tasks.

Category II employees include:

- physical therapists
- physical therapist assistants
- occupational therapists
- speech therapists
- medical social workers

Employee Exposure Category III

Category III employees perform tasks that involve no exposure to blood, body
fluids, or tissues, and Category I tasks are not a condition of their employment.
The normal work routine involves no exposure to blood, body fluids, or tissues

(although situations can be imagined or hypothesized under which anyone, anywhere, might encounter potential exposure to body fluids). Persons who perform these duties are not called upon as part of their employment to perform or assist in emergency medical care or first aid or to be potentially exposed in some other way. Tasks that involve handling of implements or utensils, use of public or shared bathroom facilities or telephones, and personal contacts such as handshaking are Category III tasks.

Category III employees include:

- administrative staff
- office staff

Employee Exposure Procedures

Now that the employee categories are established, it is important to note that training and other staff responsibilities will differ depending on the category in which an employee falls. For example, if a Category III employee is the staffing coordinator, he or she may never come in face-to-face contact with a client. However, this employee does come in contact with nurses and other caregivers who see clients. The possibility exists, therefore, that if the staff coordinator contracts tuberculosis, this infection could be passed to a nurse, who could then infect a client.

Therefore, every employee should be required to have an annual physical examination. This examination could be a health screening for which the agency identifies the specific information required, such as a tuberculosis skin test.

If any employee contracts an infection that is potentially transmissible or is exposed to an illness that leads to a period during which infection may be spread, the agency's responsibility to prevent the spread of infection to clients and other personnel may sometimes require that these persons be excluded from direct client contact or other restrictions may apply.

Persons with signs and symptoms of potentially transmissible conditions who have responsibilities for client care should report promptly to their supervisor. A sample form is provided for this purpose. Employees in this situation should complete an infection control report (see Exhibit 12–1) for further follow-up, including resumption of work duties.

INFECTION CONTROL MONITORING (SURVEILLANCE)

Infection control monitoring and surveillance activities should be done on a routine basis to ensure that staff members are conforming to uniform precautions and to ascertain whether training has had its desired effect. Additionally, the

Exhibit 12–1 Personnel Infection Control Report

Branch _____

Employee Name _____   Date _____

Symptoms/Diagnosis _____

_____ Date of Onset _____

Physician _____ Date of Visit _____

Physician Recommendations: _____

_____

_____

_____

Lab (as appropriate)_____

Approval to Return to Work (Date)_____
(Must have written consent of physician)

Special Assignment of Staff as Appropriate _____

Length of Time Unable to Work: From _____   To _____

Total Number of Working Days during This Time Period _____

Comments _____

_____

_____

_____

_____

Reported (if applicable) to: _____   Date _____

Branch Manager _____   Date _____

Infection Control Chairman _____   Date _____

Medical Director _____   Date _____

Source: Courtesy of Vickie Trevarthan, RN, Stone Mountain, Georgia.

implementation of an infection control program will satisfy external reviewers and will assist the agency to avoid litigation.

External Review Organizations

The Occupational Safety and Health Administration (OSHA) requires any organization providing health care to patients to also provide a safe work place or safe environment. The new proposed regulations on biological hazards will call for a risk reduction plan that will include a written infection control plan. These proposed rules will be applicable to home care agencies as well as to any other organization providing care.

Peer review organizations (PROs) also require the delivery of safe, effective, and appropriate care to patients. State licensure organizations will usually have some reference to the same general language as the PROs for the delivery of safe and effective care.

The Joint Commission on Accreditation of Healthcare Organizations (Joint Commission) has specific guidelines relative to infection control in the home care industry. The Joint Commission requires that measures be taken to prevent, identify, and control infections. In order to meet this requirement, agencies must as a minimum address the following components:

- personal hygiene
- isolation precautions
- aseptic procedures
- staff health and transmitted infections
- cleaning and sterilization of equipment

The Joint Commission also advises that staff members and the patient be advised of any precautions necessary for the care or treatment being rendered. All staff must be instructed in the importance of infection control and each person's responsibility in the success of the program. The Joint Commission also requires that a system be developed for evaluating, reporting, and maintaining records of infection related to the care of patients or the services being rendered.

Avoiding Litigation

The ability of the health care provider to substantiate that it has a vigorous infection control surveillance or monitoring program for detecting problems that might occur is thought by many attorneys to be among the most important defenses against unwarranted claims.

Liability concerning infection control practices usually falls under the following doctrines:

- *Respondeat superior*—(Let the master answer.) The agency is responsible for its staff.
- *Res ipsa loquitur*—(The thing speaks for itself.) This is related to the expert testimony requirement.

Employee Training

Employee infection control training effectiveness should be monitored by a four-dimensional process:

1. employee written examination (posthire, postinservice)
2. employee field audit (procedural)
3. client/caregiver interview (teaching)
4. documentation of infection

Employee infection control field monitoring should be done with new employees within the first 90 days, and evaluations should be done at least yearly thereafter. Infection control field audits should also be performed when a supervisor identifies a deficiency or notes a connection with client infections related to a particular employee or procedure. Sample audits are found in Chapter 11.

Many agency managers have a perception that once trained, all personnel will conform to the necessary infection control precautions. This perception was found to be invalid by the SENIC findings and still holds true today. To be effective, infection preventions and controls must be kept under scrutiny. Improved patient outcomes require that agency personnel take very seriously the entire issue of infection control and prevention.

Infection Control Surveillance/Monitoring Program

Monitoring adherence to agency policy and procedure and standards of practice in infection control is done through surveillance. When monitoring reveals noncompliance with recommended precautions, the conditions should be documented, along with the corrective action plan; that is, process changes, education, or retraining, if necessary. The quality assurance and improvement committee should be informed of all infection control audit results and corrective plans of action for approval or further recommendations.

Several different types of infection control audits are used in monitoring an effective infection control program. Examples of these appear at the end of this chapter in Exhibits 12–2 through 12–8.

The structure of the surveillance program should cover the following issues:

- defining the events or techniques to be monitored, such as catheter care, wound care, bag technique, or handwashing
- collecting the data in a consistent and objective manner
- consolidating the data into trends or patterns of practice
- analyzing the results and formulating action plans to resolve any identified problems
- deploying the resultant data to those responsible for correction
- evaluating the results of intervention (action plans)

Defining the events to be monitored is a method the agency can use to conduct its infection control program in a cost-effective manner. As stated earlier in this text, all occurrences warrant investigation. In the real world, however, this attitude is not practical. The focus of the infection control program should be patient-sensitive in order to gain as much "payback" in terms of improved care outcomes as possible. Some professionals would call this approach "surveillance by objectives" or "targeted surveillance."

For example, if the agency has a high admission rate for wound care, then an objective or goal would be to keep these patients infection free. It would follow that the process of dressing changes should be monitored in a systematic manner. The question to ask when attempting to define or narrow the focus of the infection control program is how the monitoring activity will improve the rate of infection. Any audit or other monitoring activity that cannot stand up to this test should be discontinued or redirected to improve patient outcomes. Agencies should also pay close attention to the OSHA guidelines on blood-borne pathogens as compliance is subject to review by regulatory agents.

Exhibit 12–2 Infection Control Field Audit for Handwashing—Skilled Nurse or HHA/CNA

DATE _____   BRANCH _____

SURVEYOR _____   EMPLOYEE _____

Handwashing Audit Instructions:

Observe and designate as applicable (A) or nonapplicable (N/A) each item on this audit. Total the points for all applicable items. The final score will be based on the total number of possible points.

Possible Points	*Actual Points*	
15	_____	1. Employee washes hands on entering the home, before touching the patient.
12	_____	2. Employee utilizes soap dispenser to wash hands.
12	_____	3. Employee utilizes paper towels to dry hands.
11	_____	4. Employee uses paper towel to turn the water faucet off.
20	_____	5. Employee's handwashing technique is appropriate.
15	_____	6. Employee washes hands during care as needed.
15	_____	7. Employee washes hands before leaving the home.
Total 100	_____	

Applicable
Points

_____ _____   Percentage of compliance

95%   Threshold

Comments: _____

_____

_____

_____

Source: Courtesy of Vickie Trevarthan, RN, Stone Mountain, Georgia.

Exhibit 12–3 Infection Control Field Audit for Bag Technique—Skilled Nurse or HHA/CNA

DATE _____   BRANCH _____

SURVEYOR _____   EMPLOYEE _____

Bag Technique Instructions:

Observe and designate as applicable (A) or nonapplicable (N/A) each item on this audit. Total the points for all applicable items. The final score will be based on the total number of possible points divided by the actual points received. Each staff member should obtain at least the 90th percentile on the final scores.

Possible Points	*Actual Points*	
12	_____	1. Bag contents are organized and reflect contents needed for routine patient care.
15	_____	2. Bag is clean.
12	_____	3. Soap and towels are stored in a separate compartment for accessibility.
11	_____	4. Bag is placed on paper.
15	_____	5. A "clean" and "dirty" area is designated and utilized on the paper.
15	_____	6. Equipment is cleaned before being returned to the bag.
20	_____	7. The aseptic compartment of the bag is entered *only* after handwashing.
Total 100	_____	

Applicable
Points

_____ _____   Percentage of compliance

90%   Threshold

Comments: _____

_____

_____

_____

Source: Courtesy of Vickie Trevarthan, RN, Stone Mountain, Georgia.

Exhibit 12–4 Infection Control Field Audit for Personal Protective Equipment Availability—Skilled Nurse, HHA, CNA, RPT, PTA, MSW

DATE _____   BRANCH _____

SURVEYOR _____   EMPLOYEE _____

Personal Protective Equipment Audit Instructions:

Observe and designate as applicable (A) or nonapplicable (N/A) each item on this audit. Total the points for all applicable items. The final score will be based on the total number of possible points.

Possible Points	Actual Points	
20	_____	1. Gloves are worn in accordance with universal precautions.
25	_____	2. All sharps are disposed of in a sharps disposal.
15	_____	3. Impervious gowns/aprons are utilized as indicated; if not indicated, employee has *available*.
14	_____	4. Employee has a mouthpiece *available*.
13	_____	5. Employee has a mask *available*.
13	_____	6. Employee has protective eyewear *available*.
Total 100	_____	

Applicable
Points

_____ _____   Percentage of compliance

95%   Threshold

Comments: _____

_____

_____

_____

Source: Courtesy of Vickie Trevarthan, RN, Stone Mountain, Georgia.

Exhibit 12–5 Infection Control Field Audit for Bed Bath—HHA, CNA

DATE_____   BRANCH _____

SURVEYOR _____   EMPLOYEE _____

Bed Bath Audit Instructions:

Observe and designate as applicable (A) or nonapplicable (N/A) each item on this audit. Total the points for all applicable items. The final score will be based on the total number of possible points.

Possible Points	Actual Points	
12	_____	1. Washes hands prior to procedure.
12	_____	2. Wears gloves.
10	_____	3. Arranges washcloth in mitten fashion.
12	_____	4. Washes each eye with a separate portion of the washcloth.
10	_____	5. Changes bath water after bathing each side of patient (x2).
15	_____	6. Patient or aide washes perineal area last.
10	_____	7. Patient's privacy is maintained.
9	_____	8. Cleans and stores equipment.
10	_____	9. Washes hands when finished with procedure.
Total 100	_____	

Applicable
Points

_____ _____   Percentage of compliance

90%   Threshold

Comments: _____
_____
_____
_____

Source: Courtesy of Vickie Trevarthan, RN, Stone Mountain, Georgia.

Exhibit 12–6   Evaluation of Administrative Standard Operating Procedures—Branch
Infection Control Audit for Personal Protective Equipment

BRANCH _____   SURVEYOR _____

BRANCH MANAGER _____   DATE _____

Branch Infection Control Audit Instructions:

   Each branch is to have available equipment and supplies necessary to minimize the risk
of infection with hepatitus B (HBV)/human immunodeficiency virus (HIV) and other
bloodborne pathogens. A surveillance of each branch will be performed randomly, but at
least biannually to ensure that required personal protective equipment is available.

   The supply closet(s) will be surveyed for the following items:

Possible Points	*Actual Points*	
50	_____	1. Gloves (sterile and nonsterile).
45	_____	2. Thermometer sheaths.
40	_____	3. Alcohol wipes.
30	_____	4. Masks.
25	_____	5. Eyewear shields.
20	_____	6. Face shields.
20	_____	7. Impervious gowns.
20	_____	8. Impervious aprons.
50	_____	9. Mouthpieces.
Total 300	_____	

Applicable
Points

_____   _____   Percentage of compliance

          95%   Threshold

Comments: _____

_____

_____

_____

Source: Courtesy of Vickie Trevarthan, RN, Stone Mountain, Georgia.

Exhibit 12–7 Infection Control Procedural Audit for Catheter Care—HHA/CNA

DATE _____   BRANCH _____

SURVEYOR _____   EMPLOYEE _____

Catheter Care Audit Instructions:

Observe and designate as applicable (A) or nonapplicable (N/A) each item on this audit. Total the points for all applicable items. The final score will be based on the total number of possible points.

Possible Points	*Actual Points*	
10	_____	1. Hands are washed immediately before any manipulation of the catheter site or apparatus.
10	_____	2. Catheter is properly secured with urinary drainage bag (UDB) "off" the floor and lower than the bladder level.
20	_____	3. Urine is emptied from the UDB without contaminating the drainage spigot.
10	_____	4. Gloves are worn in accordance with universal precautions.
20	_____	5. Catheter tubing is washed with soap and water.
20	_____	6. Meatal care/catheter care is provided with soap and water, unless otherwise specified.
10	_____	7. Hands are washed upon completion of procedure.
Total 100	_____	

Applicable
Points

_____   _____   Percentage of compliance

95%   Threshold

Comments: _____

_____

_____

_____

Source: Courtesy of Vickie Trevarthan, RN, Stone Mountain, Georgia.

Exhibit 12–8   Skilled Nurse Infection Control Procedural Home Audit for Wound Care or Dressing Change

Branch _____   Date _____

Nurse _____   Surveyor _____

	Possible Points	*Actual Points*
1. Wash hands.	5	
2. Open all needed supplies.	3	
3. Pour solution over 4x4s and/or swabs, if applicable.	4	
4. Put on nonsterile gloves.	5	
5. Remove old dressing and discard into container.	10	
6. Remove gloves and discard.	3	
7. Wash hands.	5	
8. Observe area for redness, edema, the amount and character of drainage, healing, and the patency of any drains or tubes.	15	
9. Put on nonsterile gloves (unless sterile procedure).	5	
10. Cleanse area with appropriate solution, if applicable.	4	
11. Apply any ointments, enzymatic debriders, etc., as ordered.	4	
12. Apply dressings as ordered (absorption, hydroactive, thin film, abdominal pad, etc.).	10	
13. Provide wound care in accordance with physician order.	10	
14. Remove gloves and discard with used materials.	3	
15. Tape dressing in place if indicated.	3	
16. Discard old dressing and gloves in closed container.	3	
17. Date and initial dressing.	3	
18. Wash hands.	5	
Total	100	

(N/A answers are not counted as part of the possible score.)

Final Score _____
Possible Score _____
Percentage of Compliance _____
Threshold 97%

Source: Courtesy of Vickie Trevarthan, RN, Stone Mountain, Georgia.

Chapter 13

Risk Management

The risk management issue is one that is overlooked or unmanaged by many agencies. Essentially, risk management is a process by which control of potential liabilities is effectively managed. Risk management is a comprehensive system through which all risks are identified, classified, evaluated, and controlled to predict, limit, and reduce future risks or losses.

What are the potential liabilities an agency faces? There are two major areas in which to concentrate:

1. risk to employees (i.e., workers' compensation)
2. risk to clients (i.e., incident reporting)

The risk management program should be designed to identify potential risks and resolve them *before* someone is injured. The key to the success of a risk management program is active staff participation. The staff must feel that incident reporting is an integral part of the quality assurance and improvement program. It should absolutely never be viewed as punitive.

For example, nurses have come to view incident reports as the process by which an error is reported to management or the quality assurance and improvement committee. This process is valid and should be continued. However, in order to achieve the goal of alleviating potential risks before someone is injured, an agency should look at changing the incident report to one that can include unusual occurrences or potential hazards.

An example might be that a nurse is in the home of an AIDS patient and finds no protective coverings in the home. In this case, the nurse should write the occurrence on a specific form (Exhibit 13–1) for the purpose of problem resolution or use the agency's standard incident or occurrence report (Exhibit 13–2). Additionally, the manager should complete the cause and corrective action form and submit it to the risk manager or quality assurance director (Exhibit 13–3).

Exhibit 13–1 Problem Identification Occurrence

Name _____ Date _____

Discipline _____ Branch _____

Specific Problem Identified _____

_____

_____

_____

_____

_____

_____

_____

_____

In your opinion, what caused this problem? _____

_____

_____

_____

_____

Do you have a recommendation to correct this problem? _____

_____

_____

_____

_____

WE SINCERELY APPRECIATE YOUR COMMITMENT TO IMPROVING THE AGENCY BY BRINGING THIS PROBLEM TO OUR ATTENTION. THANK YOU!

Would you like your name to be kept confidential? YES_____   NO_____

_____   _____
            Date   Signed

                                            _____
                                                   Branch Manager

The first example involved a potential client problem that could also affect the caregiver. Another example for problem identification would be where a staff member notices loose extension or phone cords running across an access route within the office. An employee could trip on the cord and sustain a workers' compensation injury as a result.

Exhibit 13–2 Incident Report (Unusual Occurrence)

THIS FORM MUST BE COMPLETED WITHIN 24 HOURS OF ANY PERSON'S ACCIDENT OR INCIDENT

TO: _____ , Attorney at Law   Occurrence Date _____

Time of Occurrence _____

Person Involved _____

Specific Place of Occurrence _____

Describe in Detail What Happened/Why It Happened/What Causes Were:

_____

_____

_____

_____

_____

Was person involved injured? _____ If yes, please specify and diagram location of injury:

Type of Injury: _____

_____ Laceration   _____

_____ Hematoma   _____

_____ Abrasion   _____

_____ Burn   _____

_____ None Apparent   _____

_____ Other (Specify)   _____

_____   _____

_____   _____

_____   _____

Name of Witness(es) _____

Name of Supervisor Notified: _____ Title: _____

Time Supervisor Notified: _____ AM _____ PM

Person Responsible for Incident _____ Branch/Dept: _____

****

FOR NURSING DEPARTMENT USE ONLY:

Was Physician Notified? Yes ____ No ____ Physician's Name _____

Time Physician Notified _____ AM _____ PM

Orders from Physician _____

Remarks _____

****

_____   _____
Supervisor   Date   Person Completing Report

                                  _____
                                  Date of Report

Exhibit 13–3 Incident Report Supplement—Cause and Corrective Action

Incident Report On _____   Date of Report _____

Branch _____

INCIDENT CATEGORY

Patient		*Employee* (must be accompanied with first report of injury)	
Patient Falls	____		
Medication Errors	____	Employee Falls at	
Lab Errors	____	Patient Home	
Order Violations	____	Employee Falls at Office	____
Procedural Errors	____	Car Accident	____
Policy Violations	____	Back Injury	____
Staffing Errors	____	Needlestick	____
Other (specify)	____	Other (specify)	____
_____		_____	
_____		_____	

Cause of Accident/Incident (Policy, Procedure, or Standard Violated):

_____

_____

_____

_____

_____

_____

_____

_____

Corrective Actions Implemented:

_____

_____

_____

_____

_____

_____

_____

_____

_____

_____   _____

Signature   Date

The completion of a form makes management aware of potential risks, on which it can then initiate action. All such forms should be sent routinely to the risk manager, who is a part of the quality assurance and improvement committee, for necessary follow-up.

Incident reports should be addressed to the agency's legal counsel. It is not necessary to actually mail these reports to legal counsel unless the incident will result in litigation. However, by addressing the incident report to legal counsel, the report can become protected under the attorney-client relationship and, therefore, not subject to subpoena. These reports are *never* filed in the client's medical record. Follow-up on such reports is absolutely essential. In this regard, the role of the risk manager should be examined closely.

RISK MANAGER ROLE

Large institutions usually have the financial resources to employ a full-time risk manager. However, most home care agencies do not have this type of flexibility. The risk management role, therefore, can be delegated to a current administrative employee. The employee need not be a nurse, although a medical background is helpful when dealing with incidents involving client care. Where a nurse is not the risk manager, the designated employee should have access to a qualified nurse for consultation.

The risk manager is a member of the quality assurance and improvement committee and reports a synopsis of all incidents related to both patients and employees. Additionally, the risk manager reports on problem identification occurrences and subsequent actions. The reports to the quality assurance and improvement committee should be trended in order for the committee to determine whether there is a pattern of practice in any specific category.

For example, incident categories should be established. The following are recommended:

- client incidents
- employee incidents
- problem identification

Each of these categories has separate classifications of problems that can be trended. Possible problem areas can be identified for tracking in each category.

Client Incidents

Typical patient incidents include:

1. Client falls—All incidents involving a client fall, whether an injury was sustained or not, should be reported in this area. The incidents should be

totaled for the report to the committee and compared with previous months in order to determine trending patterns as to location, discipline, times, etc.

2. Medication errors—This category should trend errors in medications from incorrect dosages (e.g., 5 mg when 10 was ordered, incorrect medication, failure to give medications at the prescribed times, etc.).

3. Lab work errors—This category is one often used when agencies have a large number of temporary nurses who see different clients. Inconsistent caregivers are prone to overlook lab work ordered infrequently, as in the case of a fasting blood sugar (FBS) every 90 days. Unless the case is managed by a consistent nurse, the lab work may not be done at the appropriate time. Another incident that should be reported under this category is if the nurse failed to report abnormal lab results to the physician.

4. Other order violations—This category is a catch-all for any other type of physician's order violation. For example, if a physician orders DuoDERM for a wound and the nurse uses OpSite, a client incident has occurred under this category. Another example using a potential error for paraprofessionals may be where a physician orders no weight bearing and the home health aide assists the client to the bathroom.

5. Policy violations—This category includes any violation of agency policy as it relates to patient care. For example, the agency may have a policy that employees cannot receive any gratuities. If an employee accepts a gift, there has been a policy violation. An example of a care-related policy would be where the agency has a policy not to administer experimental drugs and a nurse receives an order and administers the drug.

6. Procedural errors—This category is similar to policy violations in that it identifies errors committed resulting from nonconformance to agency procedures. For example, the agency has a procedure to change central line dressings every 72 hours in lieu of a physician's order specifying some other time span. The nurse notes that the physician ordered: "dressing change per protocol." The nurse, however, changed the dressing after seven days. In this example, there are two separate issues:
   • The order is unclear as to what specific protocol was to be used.
   • The assumption was to follow agency protocol, which was 72 hours as opposed to weekly.

7. Staffing errors—Some agencies do not see staffing errors as a client care incident. However, these occurrences do indeed lead to potential risks to clients. The most obvious example is where a nurse who is unfamiliar with a peripherally inserted catheter (PIC) line is sent to see a patient who requires technical procedures related to this type of line. Clearly, this is a staffing error. Another example is a physician order for dressing changes twice a day for seven days; on the fifth day, the nurse only made one visit.

8. Other—This category should cover any occurrence or incident not other-wise specified. When using a general category, it is important to be specific in identifying the problem.

Any one or all of these categories can be further divided at the discretion of the agency's risk manager.

Employee Incidents

It is important to categorize employee-related occurrences by groupings, as for patient incidents. Some examples follow:

1. Employee falls—These incidents should be tracked as to where they occur, i.e., in a client's home or property or at the agency's office or property. While these incidents will fall under workers' compensation, different insurance coverage may apply depending on the location of the fall.
2. Car accident—For home care providers, this will be the category most often used. If the employee has an auto accident while in the perform-ance of assigned duties, any resultant injury will fall under workers' compensation.
3. Back injury—This category is also used often in home care. Experience proves that home health aides (HHAs) are the most frequently injured under this category. Back injuries occur as a result of inappropriate positioning or inappropriate body mechanics. Root cause identification is necessary to correct this (or any) problem. Back belts are a good solution.
4. Needlestick—The use of this category is obvious. It is separated from others in order to be able to determine the need for additional training or the need for mechanical devices for appropriate disposal of sharp instruments.
5. Other—As in the patient incident groupings, this category serves as a catch-all for any other incident or occurrence. Specifics are necessary in order to trend this category.

Problem Identification

The risk manager should have a method for resolving and trending problems identified. Potential problems could be categorized if the agency deems this appropriate. This component can also work effectively as a peer review opportunity, but it must be understood by the staff that problems are identified for the purpose of individual staff development and not for punitive purposes, although sanctioning may become a part of the peer review group function. Identified trends are also used to improve process.

A sanction from a peer review group should be considered very serious. Action by management is a must. For example, a peer review group determines that a nurse is consistently performing substandard care. After investigation, it is determined that the nurse has a substance abuse problem. The peer review group can recommend that management terminate the nurse or the recommendation can be more humane and require enrollment in a treatment program during a leave of absence.

ROOT CAUSE IDENTIFICATION

The risk manager is the person designated by the agency to review, take corrective action, and follow up on all reported incidents or occurrences. Once an incident is reported, the risk manager will look for the *root cause* of the occurrence. Determining the root cause is not as simple as one might think. For example, an incident report comes to the risk manager reporting that a nurse stuck herself in the finger with a needle after an injection was given to a client. The risk manager knows every nurse has been taught not to recap needles; the assumption is made that the nurse in question did not follow the agency's policy or procedure in disposal of needles. Upon investigation, however, the risk manager finds that the nurse did not have in her possession a sharps disposal. Now the investigation needs to determine why this was missing.

Until the real cause is determined, down to the root cause, an appropriate corrective plan cannot be established. In the previous example, further investigation showed that the nurse was employed three months previously. This nurse was not given a sharps needle disposal, nor were any of the other nurses who were hired during this period of time. It was also found that the orientation plan for nurses did not address this issue. As a result, the risk manager established the following corrective plan:

1. Add hazardous waste disposal to the orientation plan for all new field employees.
2. Set up inservice for all current field employees on hazardous waste disposal.
3. Purchase sharps needle disposals for every nurse at the agency.
4. Include sharps disposals as routine supplies given to every new nurse employed.

As in this example, the corrective plan must address not only the one isolated incident, but also a systematic process to reduce future risks.

The identification of root causes is the most difficult of all functions in risk management. The root cause is simply the cause of the cause. The apparent cause, identified on the incident report, is almost never the real or root cause of an incident (see Figure 2–3, Chapter 2). The best technique for identifying the root cause is to keep asking why. The why question should be asked at least five times before you will approach the root cause. The risk manager should seek assistance with root cause identification until he or she becomes proficient with identification.

The third step in the processing of incidents is for the risk manager to follow up on the corrective plan. Without this crucial step, the risk management program is doomed to failure. Using the same incident, let us look at the follow-up on the corrective plan. The risk manager should make certain that the orientation program included a segment on hazardous waste disposal. The risk manager should place the completed date next to the correction. This process should follow the entire plan of correction until every item outlined has been completed with dates noted. Thereafter, incidents of employees sticking themselves with contaminated needles should significantly decrease.

If the risk manager finds that the same type of incidents continue to occur even after the corrective plan has been fully implemented, the indication would be that the root cause on the initial incident was incorrectly stated. It cannot be emphasized strongly enough that the root cause will be the determining factor in a successful risk management program.

The risk manager who is having difficulty determining root causes should consult the quality assurance and improvement committee. The collective wisdom of the committee can sometimes find the root cause of incidents more easily than someone working too closely with the problem.

All managers are interested in results. The end result of an effective risk management program is called *loss ratio* for workers' compensation and *occurrence ratio* for patient incidents. The board of directors or senior management of the agency must make a determination of the acceptable level of risk to the company.

WORKERS' COMPENSATION LOSS RATIO

The workers' compensation loss ratio is a mechanism the risk manager can use to determine whether the agency's losses in the employee incident category are within an acceptable range and to continuously improve the range. The loss ratio is calculated using the following formula:

Total Benefits Paid ÷ Total Gross Wages = Loss Ratio

Let's say that we want to determine the agency's loss ratio for the first quarter of 1993. Total salaries for the three months were $457,526. Total benefits paid out by workers' compensation, including wages for lost work days, were $4,396. Applying the formula:

$$\$4,396 \div \$457,526 = .0096 \text{ (loss ratio percentage)}$$

Less than 1 percent is an outstanding loss ratio for any agency. However, most agencies have higher ratios. Again, the board should determine an acceptable ratio for the agency based on a historical perspective of the issue and should begin continuous quality improvements to reduce the ratio.

There are many ways the risk manager can influence this ratio. The most important is to get employees back to work after an injury as quickly as possible. Second medical opinions are helpful when an injury has been sustained. The employee's case should be managed in the same manner as any other client under the care of the agency. The agency's best assurance of low loss ratios is the appointment of an official workers' compensation physician. All employees with work-related injuries should be required to see an agency-appointed physician who believes in returning employees to work as soon as possible. This physician is not paid by the agency; rather, he or she is paid by the workers' compensation carrier when an employee goes for treatment.

It should be noted that most agencies that have a cost control program for the aggressive management of workers' compensation claims have concentrated solely on controlling claim costs. Controlling costs after an injury is beneficial but inadequate in today's competitive marketplace. Claims costs should be prevented, not just controlled. This forms the basis for the entire continuous quality improvement movement. The majority of these costs can be prevented if and when root cause identification is coupled with an aggressive process correction. Inadequate process is the largest contributor to spiraling workers' compensation claims.

OCCURRENCE RATIO

The occurrence ratio for patient incidents works similarly to the loss ratio. The occurrence ratio answers the question: "What percentage of patients does the agency expect to be incident-free?"

Again, the board of directors should answer this question based on a historical perspective of the agency's incidents. The reader should be cautioned that this percentage should have flexibility; in that, the goal of risk management is to encourage incident reporting in order to correct current problems and minimize future risks. If the percentage of occurrence ratio is set too low, caregivers and managers alike will feel the pressure not to report minor occurrences.

While everyone would like to believe that 100 percent of clients will be incident-free, 100 percent of the time, this is not realistic. Caregivers are not perfect, and mistakes will be made. Each mistake, however, offers the risk manager an opportunity to facilitate the improvement of overall care rendered by the agency. The occurrence ratio formula follows:

Number of Incidents ÷ Unduplicated Census = Occurrence Ratio

An example of the formula is:

26 Incidents ÷ 837 Patients = .03 Occurrence Ratio

The risk manager should review closely any office that does not have any incidents. The risk manager needs to be aware that setting the occurrence ratio too low can have an adverse effect on incident reporting and consequently should monitor closely those who never report an incident.

TRENDING

Throughout this chapter, trending has been emphasized. The process of trending is simply a statistically valid grouping of incidents by type, person, time, age of client, or employee. This trending will enable the risk manager to establish a patient risk profile and an employee risk profile that will identify and assist management in the prediction and reduction of future incidents.

For example, the risk manager may identify that, over a three-month period, 40 percent of client incidents involved falls. Of that group, 70 percent occurred while an HHA was ambulating the client. Additionally, the risk manager may identify that 98 percent of the client falls occurred in clients over the age of 70. While specific problems can be resolved without trending, this root cause would be hard to identify without the accumulation of data through the trending process.

In this example, the root cause can be identified as failure to adequately train HHAs in safely ambulating patients over age 70. As mentioned previously, the root cause must be identified accurately prior to initiating an action plan to not only resolve the problem but also to prevent its recurrence.

The risk manager has many other duties to oversee. He or she should also be responsible for compliance with the Occupational Safety and Health Act (OSHA), which requires at least an annual report to the federal government. In this regard, this employee should check periodically the physical locations of each office to ensure employee safety. The risk manager also should be aware of and comply with fire laws and be responsible for disaster plans. For home care, a disaster plan could cover impassable roads, violent and destructive weather, earthquakes, power outages, etc.

While most home care agencies do not have a risk manager, this functional area of responsibility is a must. Risk management is too important to the overall survival of an agency and far too important to improved quality to allow these responsibilities to become fragmented among several people.

JOINT COMMISSION REQUIREMENTS

The Joint Commission on Accreditation of Healthcare Organizations (Joint Commission) has several requirements that apply to risk management. These include safety measures utilized in the home to minimize risks to patients and caregivers. Safety, which is strongly emphasized, relates to the education of patients in basic home safety, safe use of medical equipment, storage and use of supplies, and any relevant precautions necessary to care and treatment. The Joint Commission further requires that safety management, infection control, and emergency preparedness plans be monitored and evaluated along with the patient's knowledge regarding all safety factors affecting his or her care. Staff knowledge and performance of safe and effective use of equipment is also a requirement.

How many times have you seen the statement, "remove scatter rugs" under the safety measures of a plan of treatment? This type of "pat answer" to safety requirements is not adequate. The safety requirements should be diagnosis specific and address the individualized needs of the patient.

CONCEPTS FOR RISK MANAGEMENT

- Risk identification is accomplished through collecting data from any and all of the following sources:
  1. incident reporting
  2. occurrence reporting
  3. workers' compensation claims
  4. safety checks at physical locations
  5. OSHA reports
  6. external audit/survey reports
  7. attorney requests for records
  8. patient complaints
  9. reimbursements or settlements
- Risk analysis is the evaluation of the data to determine the effect of risks and the prevention strategy to minimize those risks. Analysis may include:
  1. root cause identification
  2. trending
  3. statistical methods

- Risk control is the plan to correct problems that pose risks to the agency. Correction plans should be process oriented and prevention driven. This area of risk management will also include claim cost control measures.
- Risk financing comes into play when the risk to the agency cannot be prevented, controlled, avoided, or shifted. Risk financing requires an evaluation of the agency's risk exposure and a determination of what risks (if any) the agency is willing to finance (risk retention) versus those risks the agency insures against (risk transfer).

MEETING PATIENT EXPECTATIONS

Patients who complain are a potential risk to the agency. This risk may be one of lost revenue or one of potential litigation. In either event, the risk manager needs to be aware of complaints and able to address their root causes to prevent them from recurring.

A study by the Coca-Cola Company found that for every complaint a company gets, there are 26 other unhappy people who did not voice their complaint. If these numbers can be believed, we can multiply every complaint by 26. How does this affect patient satisfaction results? The risk manager should work closely with the customer service department to ensure that all complaints are identified and root causes found.

Many agency managers will voluntarily refund money to a client who is not satisfied with care or will make some other monetary adjustment. As with patient complaints, these occurrences should be monitored to identify root causes, which will lead to process changes necessary to prevent recurrences. The patient refund policy is an excellent way to track these types of problems. It will assist the agency in "getting its priorities straight."

All attorney inquiries should be routinely referred to the risk manager for handling. These inquiries are potential red flags for the risk manager to monitor carefully. These, like all other issues in risk management, should be trended and statistically analyzed.

Consistently meeting the expectations and needs of patients is what the continuous quality improvement program is all about. This chapter has shown negative consequences to the agency when those needs are not met. If the agency is to stay in business, preventing risks is of utmost importance.

Chapter 14

Administration and Operational Review

Administrative review audits are as varied as the different types of agencies in the nation. The purpose and scope of these audits also vary depending on the agency's priorities. These audits are especially helpful when the agency has multiple branch locations.

In the home care industry, the end product is largely controlled by the person rendering the care. There can be no automation of service delivery. In a McDonald's, for example, you get the same Big Mac regardless of where in the world you order it. Service providers are not able to automate to this extent. However, policy, procedures, and standards are a method by which the concepts of automation can occur. These rules by which care is rendered are known as quality control measures.

For example, an initial visit should be made within 24 hours of receiving a physician's order to start care. When the agency states this criterion as a policy, it becomes automated. Every patient in every branch should be seen within 24 hours.

Administrative review audits are designed to test the agency or branch on the established criteria set forth as policy or procedures. Additionally, since customer satisfaction is a determination of quality, questionnaires designed to gauge the degree to which patients are satisfied with care are essential. Finally, questionnaires designed to determine staff satisfaction should also be a part of the administrative review.

THE BRANCH AUDIT

The most prevalent administrative review audit is the branch audit. The four main components of this type of surveillance tool are the purpose, the scope, the indicators, and the thresholds.

Purpose

The purpose of the branch audit is to determine compliance with corporate policy, procedures, and standards by monitoring major functional areas of responsibility. A multilocation agency can use this audit tool to ensure consistency of operations. A single location agency can use the tool to ensure that processes are in place to support policy and procedure.

Scope

The audit's scope is the functional areas of responsibility of key personnel over the previous six (or twelve) months.

Indicators

Indicators are as follows:

- Branch Manager
  1. Growth
  2. Profitability
  3. Audit results of director of professional services and staffing coordinators
  4. Risk management:
     (a) Workers' compensation loss ratio
     (b) Patient incidents occurrence ratio
  5. Customer satisfaction ratings
- Director of Professional Services (DPS):
  1. Audit results of quality assurance and utilization review
  2. Denial rates
  3. Field staff turnover rates
  4. Nonadmitted patients and reasons
  5. Personnel qualifications
  6. Visit limitations by payer source
- Staffing Coordinator (SC) or Office Manager:
  1. Productivity ratios of field staff
  2. Collection period ratios
  3. Missed visits
  4. Consistent caregivers
  5. Medical records format
  6. Care starts within standard

Unlike the clinical indicators that look at structure, process, and outcomes, the indicators for an administrative audit review the structure in an office for outcomes. These indicators are all set by the corporation in policy, procedure, or standard. Therefore, the other two categories of indicators are unnecessary.

Thresholds

The thresholds for administrative audits are also unlike those of the diagnosis-related quality assurance audits in that these thresholds are stated in terms of expectations or specifications of the corporation, and they are designed to be results or outcome oriented. For example, the expectation or standard for growth could be 10 percent over the previous review period. Examples of thresholds for the branch audit follow:

- Branch Manager:
  1. Growth—10 percent over previous six (or twelve) months
  2. Profitability—8 percent of net revenue year-to-date
  3. Audit results:
     (a) DPS: Combined audit results of 80 percent
     (b) SC: Combined audit results of 80 percent
  4. Risk management:
     (a) Workers' compensation: Loss ratio of 5 percent of gross salaries
     (b) Patient incidents: 5 percent of unduplicated census year-to-date
  5. Customer satisfaction—Returned questionnaires with 98 percent satisfaction
- Director of Professional Services:
  1. Audits:
     (a) QA audits: Combined results of 85 percent
     (b) UR audits: Combined results of 90 percent
  2. Denial rates: no greater than 2.4 percent of visits billed to Medicare
  3. Turnover rates: no greater than 8 percent of staff by discipline
  4. Nonadmits: 99 percent meet nonadmit criteria
  5. Personnel qualifications: 98 percent meet compliance standard
- Staffing Coordinators:
  1. Productivity ratios:
     (a) Level I RN: 35 visits per week
     (b) Level II RN (Case Managers): 25 visits per week
     (c) Level III RN (Clinical Specialist): 15 visits per week
     (d) HHA: 30 visits per week
  2. Collection period ratios—45 days

3. Missed visits—98 percent compliance to orders
4. Consistent caregivers—85 percent consistency
5. Medical records format—95 percent compliance
6. Care started within time frame—98 percent conformance

These thresholds demonstrate that the administrative audit is a culmination of all the outcomes of the key personnel in each office. The combined point score percentage gives the overall result of compliance by job categories.

The quantification of review results allows objectivity in the evaluation of personnel and ties performance-based criteria to quality outcomes. Continuous quality improvement methods for process control charts will allow individuals to track their own performance over time. Individuals also will be able to determine whether a process is "in control" and whether the process or function is capable of meeting the threshold requirements. If not, the process manager must improve the way in which the process functions before improved performance can result.

It cannot be overemphasized that the methods of continuous quality improvement are intended to make management aware that the root cause of problems affecting performance outcomes is generally (94 percent of the time) the process rather than an individual's fault.

It is the responsibility of management to correct process problems, not the responsibility of people who work in the process. Mid-level managers who are accountable for a specific process should be empowered to improve the process with the help of subordinates. Without this type of empowerment, the continuous quality improvement methods will be of little use in bringing about the changes necessary to produce sustained improvements. A sample audit for administration follows in Exhibit 14–1.

The branch audit may appear to be simple and encompass few questions. It should be reiterated here that the quality assurance and improvement program is designed to cover all relevant issues on the overall operation and functioning of an agency, but does not duplicate effort. Again, agencies have neither the time nor the financial resources for duplicative work. The branch audit purpose is to review the results of major areas of functional responsibility, not to audit individual records. For example, the office manager or staffing coordinator is tested on collection period ratio at the company standard of 45 days. This standard takes into consideration timely billing and all collection efforts. It is, therefore, unnecessary to ask questions pertaining to billing. To figure this ratio, use the following formulas:

a. Total Net Revenue ÷ Workdays in Period = Average Sales per Day
b. Outstanding Accounts Receivable ÷ Average Sales Every Day = Average Collection Days Ratio

Exhibit 14–1 Administrative Review Branch Audit

Branch _____ Date _____

Branch Manager _____

Director of Professional Services _____

Office Manager _____

Possible Points	*Actual Points*	**PART I: BRANCH MANAGER**
		1. Total visits first 6 months _____
		Total visits previous 6 months _____
		Total revenue first 6 months _____
		Total revenue previous 6 months _____
_15_	_____	Percentage of +/– visits _____ Threshold _10%_
		Met _____ Not Met _____
_15_	_____	Percentage of +/– revenue _____ Threshold _10%_
		Met _____ Not Met _____
		Data Source: Financial Statements
_30_	_____	2. Profitability Y-T-D Current Period _____ Threshold _8%_
		Met _____ Not Met _____
		Data Source: Financial Statements
_20_	_____	3. Number of Patient Questionnaires Returned _____
		Positive _____ Satisfaction % _____
		Threshold _98%_ Met _____ Not Met _____
		Data Source: All Patient Questionnaires
_20_	_____	4. Number of Physician Questionnaires Returned _____
		Positive _____ Satisfaction % _____
		Threshold _98%_ Met _____ Not Met _____
		Data Source: All Physician Questionnaires
_20_	_____	5. Workers' Compensation Benefits Paid _____
		Total Direct Gross Salary _____ Loss Ratio % _____
		Threshold _2.5%_ Met _____ Not Met _____
		Data Source: Insurance Company Statistics and Financial Statements
_20_	_____	6. Unemployment Compensation Benefits Paid _____
		Total Gross Salary _____ Loss Ratio % _____
		Threshold _2.5%_ Met _____ Not Met _____
		7. Total # of Patient Incidents Reported: _____ Of the incidents reported:
_15_	_____	a. Was the root cause correctly identified?
		Correct Root Cause % _____ Threshold _80%_
		Met _____ Not Met _____
_15_	_____	b. Was the corrective plan implemented?
		Implemented % _____ Threshold _90%_
		Met _____ Not Met _____
_25_	_____	8. Results Part II DPS _____
		Threshold _80%_ Met _____ Not Met _____

Exhibit 14–1 continued

Possible Points	*Actual Points*	
25		9. Results Part III Officer Manager/Staffing Coordinator _____ Threshold _80%_ Met _____ Not Met _____ Data Source: Results of Current Branch Audit
220		% Compliance _____ Threshold _____85%_____

_____	_____
Reviewer	Branch Manager

_____
Reviewer

PART II: DIRECTOR OF PROFESSIONAL SERVICES

Possible Points	*Actual Points*	

20		1. QA audit results from all previous audits in 6 month period:
		  a. Diagnosis-related audits combined results _____
		    Threshold _____85%_____ Met _____ Not Met _____

20		b. Service audits combined results _____ Threshold _____85%_____ Met _____ Not Met _____

20		c. UR audits combined results _____ Threshold ___90%__
		                           Met _____ Not Met _____
		  Data Source: All audits for 6 months
		2. Total billed visits previous quarter _____
		  Total denied visits _____

10		Denial rate % _____ Threshold __2%__ Met _____ Not Met _____ Data Source: Intermediary Denials/Financial Statements for units

10		3. a. Staff turnover rates: Total RN positions _____
		    # RN terminated _____
		    RN turnover rate % _____ Threshold _10%_
		                           Met _____ Not Met _____

10		b. Staff turnover rates: Total HHA positions _____
		    # HHA terminated _____
		    HHA turnover rate % _____ Threshold _10%__
		                           Met _____ Not Met _____
		Data Source: Staff positions determined by Master Schedules
		for 6 months (exclude employees who have moved or retired)
		4. Is progressive counseling evident when indicated by:

10		a. Inservice attendance % _____ Threshold _100%_ Met _____ Not Met _____ Data Source: Inservice attendance slip in personnel folder
10		b. Work attendance % _____ Threshold _100%_ Met _____ Not Met _____ Data Source: Updated calendar of absenteeism
10		c. Paperwork submission within deadlines % _____ Threshold _100%_ Met _____ Not Met _____ Data Source: Office Manager's Late Paperwork Listing

continues

Exhibit 14–1 continued

Possible Points	*Actual Points*	
		5. Personnel qualifications: Total # of Professional Staff ____ Total HHA ____
20	_____	a. Licenses on professional staff: _____ % _____ Threshold 100% Met ____ Not Met ____
10	_____	b. Physicals: Total Staff _____ Evidence of physicals _____ % _____ Threshold 100% Met ____ Not Met ____
10	_____	c. References: Total Staff _____ Evidence of references _____ % _____ Threshold 100% Met ____ Not Met ____
10	_____	d. Evaluations: Total Staff _____ Evidence of evaluations _____ % _____ Threshold 100% Met ____ Not Met ____
		6. Nonadmitted patients: Total # of nonadmits _____ Total # should have been admitted _____
10	_____	Nonadmit ratio % _____ Threshold 99% Met ____ Not Met ____ Data Source: Nonadmits previous 6 months
		7. Medical Record Standards Compliance: Census _____ Records Reviewed _____
10	_____	a. HHA SV notes: Documented every 14 days _____ Threshold 100% Met ____ Not Met ____
10	_____	b. Patient care conference: Documented every 30 days _____ Threshold 100% Met ____ Not Met ____
10	_____	c. Clinical record reviews: Documented every 60 days _____ Threshold 100% Met ____ Not Met ____
10	_____	d. Signed POT within 7 days _____ Threshold 100% Met ____ Not Met ____
10	_____	e. Care plans updated every 30 days _____ Threshold 80% Met ____ Not Met ____ Data Source: 10% random sample of current records
230	_____	Total Amount _____% Threshold 85% Met ____ Not Met ____

_____   _____
Reviewer   Director of Professional Services

_____
Reviewer

Exhibit 14–1 continued

Possible Points	Actual Points	

Possible Points / *Actual Points*

PART III: OFFICE MANAGER/STAFFING COORDINATOR

1. Productivity Ratio Compliance:

10 _____   a. Level I RNs
Total # of workdays _____ × 7 = _____
                         Met _____ Not Met _____
Total visits made _____

10 _____   b. Level II RNs
Total # of workdays _____ × 2 = _____
Clinical Coordinator
Total # of workdays _____ × 5 = _____ Case Manager
                         Met _____ Not Met _____
Total # of workdays _____ × 3 = _____
Start of care only or 7 routine visits
Total visits made _____

10 _____   c. Level III RNs
Total # of workdays _____ × 3 = _____
                         Met _____ Not Met _____
Total visits made _____

10 _____   d. HHAs
Total # of workdays _____ × 6.6 = _____
                         Met _____ Not Met _____
Total visits made _____
Data Source: Productivity Report × 3 months

2. Collection Period Ratios:

5 _____   a. Medicare _____ Threshold 28 days
                         Met _____ Not Met _____
15 _____   b. Medicaid _____ Threshold 45 days
                         Met _____ Not Met _____
20 _____   c. Private _____ Threshold 45 days
                         Met _____ Not Met _____
Data Source: Aging Report

3. Visits in Accordance with Physician Orders?
20 _____   Total visits ordered _____ Threshold 95%
                         Met _____ Not Met _____
Total visits made in accordance with the order _____
Total visits made not in accordance with the order _____
Data Source: Randomly select 20 records, see most frequent
order/compare to previous months' visits in record

4. Consistent Caregivers:
10 _____   RN consistent visits _____ RN inconsistent visits _____
10 _____   HHA consistent visits _____ HHA inconsistent visits _____
RN consistent caregivers % _____ Threshold 80%
                         Met _____ Not Met _____
HHA consistent caregivers % _____ Threshold 80%
                         Met _____ Not Met _____

continues

Exhibit 14–1 continued

Possible Points	Actual Points	
		Data Source: Same 20 records as #3—count all visits for total—count consistent care (i.e., same RN or HHA) and count inconsistent caregiver visits. DO NOT COUNT WEEKENDS/ CONSULT VISITS/EVENING/START OF CARE (SOC)
		5. Medical Records
5	_____	a. Format? # of records not accurate _____
		Threshold _90%_ _____% Met _____ Not Met _____
10	_____	b. Timely? # of records not filed timely _____
		Threshold _90%_ _____% Met _____ Not Met _____
		Data Source: Same 20 records—any record not in format or not filed timely is counted against universe
		6. Turnaround Times for Discrepancy within Guidelines?
5	_____	RN within 24 hours of evaluation date—# of records not within time _____
		Threshold _95%_ _____% Met _____ Not Met _____
5	_____	HHA within 48 hours of SOC—# of records not within time
		Threshold _95%_ _____% Met _____ Not Met _____
5	_____	Therapy within 72 hours of SOC—# of records not within time _____
		Threshold _95%_ _____% Met _____ Not Met _____
		Data Source: Same 20 records
150	_____	% Compliance _____ Threshold _85%_

_____ _____
Reviewer Office Manager

_____
Reviewer

POT = plan of treatment; PTF = personnel transaction form; SV = skilled visit; Y-T-D = year-to-date.

THE RESULTS-ORIENTED AUDIT

In order for a branch or agency to do well on a results-oriented audit, process or procedures to ensure the expected outcomes must be followed. If expected outcomes are not achieved, the methods of continuous quality improvement should be employed to determine whether the process is capable of producing the desired results. The results-oriented audit shortcuts the process for procedure auditing, yet achieves the same expectations.

This type of results-oriented audit is similar to other audit types in that it identifies the data source from which the information should be obtained and is so objective in nature that anyone conducting the survey would have the same result. In single branch agencies, the administrator could conduct the survey for the director of professional services and the office manager. It is recommended that the chair of the board or the person to whom the branch manager reports conduct the branch audit for the administrator.

In multibranch operations, it is recommended that in addition to the branch manager conducting this audit process, the regional staff also do so periodically. It is strongly suggested that each person holding a key position be given the audit tool to use as a guide and working model to know the standards by which he or she will be judged and the methods of continuous quality improvement to track their results.

Employees can conduct this audit on themselves and their processes and gain a feeling of security when they know the criteria by which they will be evaluated. The audit tool also helps to focus employees on those issues that are most important to the agency.

One of the biggest opportunities for improvement that managers face is the ability to focus staff on the key issues that affect the quality and reimbursement of service. The administrative audits are designed to help managers meet this growing challenge.

JOINT COMMISSION REQUIREMENTS

The administrative requirements under the Joint Commission on Accreditation of Healthcare Organizations (Joint Commission) are numerous. Every administrator should order the most recently revised edition of the home care standards for accreditation put out by the Joint Commission for study and review.

A summary of the most important administrative requirements is provided below.

Patient Rights and Responsibilities

These standards deal primarily with the patient's right of informed consent and decision making regarding his or her care. In this regard, the agency has the responsibility to inform the client of all procedures and actions before they take place and to ensure that understanding is acknowledged. If the agency serves populations of non-English-speaking clients, arrangements should be made for interpreters. Likewise, arrangements should be made to assure that the deaf and illiterate understand the information provided.

Patients have the right to report a grievance without repercussions (this is also a professional review organization [PRO] requirement). The agency must respect the clients' decisions regarding care and treatment or their refusal of treatment.

Management and Administration

These standards address the overall management of the agency by a qualified individual who takes steps to ensure compliance with applicable laws, regulatory organizations, and inspection groups. The administrator or branch manager is responsible for implementing all policies and procedures approved by the board of directors. Policies and procedures regarding the service delivery component are developed with the assistance of appropriate professionals and go through periodic review.

Lines of responsibility and accountability are clearly established. There are written personnel policies and procedures that are implemented.

Financial management follows policy and procedure. For any service not provided directly, there is a written contract.

Governing Body

The governing body has the legal authority for the agency. The board communicates with the administration of the agency in a systematic manner. There is an operating budget in compliance with applicable law approved by the board. This group also appoints the administrator of the agency via procedure. There is a process approved by the board to ensure that all personnel providing care are competent and qualified.

The board receives, at least annually, reports on the quality and appropriateness of patient care and the allocation of resources. With these and other reports, the board annually evaluates the agency's performance. When there are multiple locations, the board will also delineate the level of authority to each.

A conflict-of-interest policy is in place and implemented for all board decisions, and members have the responsibility to perform their duties as prescribed in the policies and procedures of the agency.

MEDICAL RECORDS ADMINISTRATION

Home care is an industry that has survived its infancy and is now going through puberty. The industry, which has not matured sufficiently to produce a reliable acuity system, also has not matured to the point that medical records administration is given the support necessary for a professional system.

These industry failings notwithstanding, the management of the medical record is of primary importance to the quality program. Many functions of medical records administration are currently being performed by several people. For example, agencies generally have a clerk responsible for filling in the medical record. Someone is also designated to review the discharge record for completeness. In many agencies, this review is accomplished by a nurse when it is really no more than a clerical review procedure. The protection of records is generally assumed to be a task of the director of professional services or the administrator rather than of a medical records technician. The director of professional services, who has many issues to juggle, generally does not give top priority to patient privacy issues when information is requested or received.

Nurses or others at an agency often are unable to locate a medical record. Countless time is then wasted while staff run all over the agency searching for the record. Sooner or later it turns up, but never at the opportune moment. The result of these scenarios is that valuable resources are wasted on tasks that could better be handled at a lower level, in a more comprehensive way. The issue is one of focus. If one person at the agency has the responsibility for medical records administration, the performance of the job will improve. Common responsibilities found under the broad title of medical records administration are discussed below.

Filing

The largest expenditure of time in medical records administration is for the filing of documents in the record. Until the utopian time when every agency has the capability to computerize all medical records, filing will be necessary. Large volume agencies sometimes fall behind in filing. Patient care suffers when this is allowed to continue over an extended period of time. Caregivers need to have up-to-date information in the medical record to manage the care properly. Caregivers consequently must turn in their documentation in a timely manner. The federal Conditions of Participation require documentation to be in the medical record within seven days. The following procedure usually occurs:

- Caregivers do not all come into the office on a daily basis but are generally required to turn in documentation at least weekly.
- Once the documentation comes in, it generally goes through some type of review.
- Appropriate documentation is then given to medical records for filing.

Given this course of events, it is unrealistic to believe the agency will ever be in compliance with the requirements to file within seven days. Obviously, the agency cannot allow itself to be out of compliance, nor is it realistic to believe this requirement will be changed. The only course of action for the agency is to use continuous quality improvement techniques to improve the process.

Storage and Retrieval of Records

Most agencies file records by patient name. Some file by payer source or at least have some type of color-coded label for payer identification. Numerical filing, which is used by some agencies, was used extensively in the 1970s. These systems are limited and offer the biggest challenge in repeat admissions. Most agencies open a new record whenever a patient is readmitted after a certain time period. This does not allow the agency access to the historical data that have been accumulated over time.

This issue also involves the confusion over unduplicated census count. Many agencies ignore the requirements of unduplicated census because the retrieval system is not sensitive enough to track admissions. Duplicates are therefore counted as new admissions.

Terminal digit systems allow a historical record to be utilized for all admissions. This type of state-of-the-art system should be considered by large volume agencies.

Record Tracking

Tracking systems for medical records are a must for large volume agencies and those with problems finding records in a timely manner. These systems can be computerized or manual, simple or complex, depending on the needs of the agency. A tracking system minimally should have a card in the place of a missing file with a designation as to where the file can be located. The medical records technician should have the ability to check out all medical records and know exactly where records are at any given time.

Some problems with these systems:

- Once the record is checked out, the nurse may loan the record to someone else, negating the entire system.
- Someone could bypass the medical records technician with the excuse "I'll only be a minute." Minutes stretch into hours.

When setting up a tracking system, these "failure points" should be considered.

Analysis of the Record

Upon discharge of the patient, the medical records technician should organize the record into such form and format as the agency deems appropriate for storage and possible later retrieval. During this process, the technician should utilize a simple checksheet to determine the completeness of the record and the data elements that are missing. This is strictly a quantitative analysis for the purpose of identifying those portions of the medical record that are incomplete, e.g., signatures, discharge summary, etc.

The qualitative analysis process, which identifies problems or inaccuracies in the documentation, should be done by a nurse. This type of review is outside the scope of the medical records function.

Another type of analysis that could be performed by the medical records technician is the statistical analysis. This analysis can abstract certain data elements for use in the overall quality assurance and improvement program. Examples include:

- By diagnosis, how many visits, by which disciplines, occurred during the course of treatment?
- How many visits on the average were made to all patients by payer source?
- What is the average length of stay?
- Does length of stay vary by diagnosis or other intervening variables such as age, sex, and presence or absence of significant other?

This type of information can be extremely valuable in the quality assurance studies and in the development of screening methods for "outlier determination."

Certain states have statistical data-gathering requirements under the state's health planning organization. The medical records technician can supply these data on an ongoing basis as well. This type of data generally seeks to identify the total number of patients served by county, ethnic mix, age, etc.

Administrative and Clinical Support Functions

The medical records technician should have the responsibility to protect records and maintain the confidential nature of client information. All personnel of an agency have the ethical responsibility to protect the confidential nature of information imparted to them. The medical records technician, however, should be delegated the overall responsibility of ensuring that medical information is never placed where it will be visible to a passerby, that client names are not posted in any manner, etc.

Protecting the privacy of clients extends to releases of information to other health care facilities, payers, review organizations, etc. A central person should be vested with the latest knowledge of these issues and be prepared to offer recommendations to the administrator on changes in policy and procedure regarding the latest technology. For example, with the wide use of the facsimile (FAX) machine in today's business environment, policies and procedures should be amended to state whether the agency will allow patient information to be transmitted in this unguarded fashion.

Note that the discussion of release of information did not mention attorneys. As discussed previously, all correspondence regarding patients from or to attorneys should be directed through the risk manager.

Joint Commission Requirements Regarding the Medical Record

The Joint Commission discusses the home care records in its standards for accreditation. In brief, these standards are:

- An accurate medical record is maintained covering all services rendered to the patient and responses to treatment.
- A standardized format is used in the record for documenting all care.
- The agency has policies covering who may make entries in and review the medical record.
- A standard explanatory legend defines any abbreviations used in the medical record.
- Discharge records are completed within a reasonable period of time.
- Length of time for maintenance of clinical records is recorded in policy and procedure and is in accordance with applicable law.
- Reasonable security measures are taken to protect the records from unauthorized use, and patient care confidentiality is maintained.

Issues of medical records administration obviously should be given their proper place in the hierarchy of agency affairs. Agency administrators will need to give considerable thought to the level of staff person employed in this position. Certification courses are available for those desiring to learn more about the professional components of medical records administration and management.

As home care agencies continue to improve services and the quality of those services, it follows that administrative services will require improvements as well. Total quality management seeks to look at every aspect of the agency to find areas for improvements.

Being good is no longer good enough in today's competitive market.

Chapter 15

Staff Development

The importance of staff development has been discussed throughout this book. Aggressive staff development is the key element in attaining quality assurance and continuous improvement. Staff development, like many other important components in the home care program, is often unfocused. All too often, staff development needs are determined by whomever happens to be available to present an inservice or other program. All too often agencies see the inservices as just another rule with which conformance is mandatory under the federal Conditions of Participation.

Developing the staff of an agency, like any other worthwhile task, requires a plan. This plan should have the same goal as the quality assurance and improvement program, e.g., improved outcomes of care. This goal can be examined in relation to the orientation of new nurses.

NURSE ORIENTATION OVERVIEW

Nurse orientation includes the following goals and objectives:

1. Teach new nurses the concept of case management versus visits for technical procedures.
   - Objective: Teach nurses to identify and intervene with total client needs, e.g., socioeconomic/environmental problems could complicate client's condition and interfere with expected outcomes. Care planning is the process to be mastered.
   - Outcome: Improved care when nurses apply case management principles in care planning.
2. Teach new nurses that the client record is a reflection of their practice.
   - Objective: Teach nurses the theories and practical application of total chart documentation in conformance with established agency policies and procedures and external review requirements.

- Outcome: Appropriate charting allows for ease in case management and supervisory oversight and also identifies unresolved client problems for further intervention, i.e., improved outcomes.
3. Teach new nurses community-based resources to meet client needs and methods of access.
    - Objective: Teach nurses when and how to use available resources to augment primary care.
    - Outcome: Improved patient care when all resources work cooperatively.
4. Teach new nurses the concepts of customer service.
    - Objective: Health care professionals have never been acclimated to "customer" satisfaction. The orientation should address issues concerning:
        — client and family rights and responsibilities
        — client and family involvement in care planning
        — client and family expectations regarding treatment and visit times
        — client and family right to decide their social and life styles without judgmental attitudes
    - Outcome: Nurses should meet client's expectations, i.e., quality is largely determined by the user of service.
5. Teach new nurses the practical application of theories to minimize risk to clients and themselves.
    - Objective: Teach nurses issues of client abandonment, patient abuse or negligence, assumption of risk, and issues regarding self-protection in uncontrolled environments.
    - Outcome: Improved ability to manage risks.
6. Teach new nurses qualifying criteria and coverage issues under various federal and state programs.
    - Objective: Teach nurses to move clients into and out of appropriate programs based on medical condition.
    - Outcome: Clients continue to receive needed services at the appropriate level while agency continues to receive payment.

It is important to note that the orientation classes will form an impression of the overall philosophy of the agency on all new nurses and other staff. This philosophy should be clear from the instructor that the agency is quality driven and has as its standard expected patient outcomes of care.

THE PRECEPTOR PROGRAM

Classroom instruction is only the first step of orientation for field staff. The second, and equally important step, is a preceptor program. Employees can get theory in a classroom but translating that theory into practical application requires tutelage. The preceptor program is designed to train nurses and others in the field and to reinforce expected outcomes of client care.

In order to ensure that preceptors are teaching in accordance with the prescribed curriculum, a preceptor training program is also a necessity. The preceptors must be validated prior to accepting the responsibility of training new nurses. This process also builds in standards that decrease variation. The goal is to make good habits an overlearned skill. If bad habits become overlearned, then relearning becomes extremely difficult.

The preceptor's training program should include at least the following:

1. Preceptors should achieve complete familiarity with and validation of the orientation program for new nurses.
2. Preceptors should be taught to train nurses in home care assessments, planning, intervention, and evaluation techniques.
3. Preceptors should be taught to train nurses on standards of practice in relation to the home care setting, with emphasis on outcomes by diagnosis.
4. Preceptors should be taught the techniques of chart audit.
5. Preceptors should be taught to train nurses on charting expectations.

A preceptor should be assigned to every new nurse for at least 30 days postorientation. During this time, the preceptor should review all the work of the new nurse in order to assure that good habits are being overlearned. Thereafter, the preceptor should make recommendations for the nurse in terms of further training. Depending on the type of training required, the preceptor or staff development director should meet these additional training needs.

CIRCUMVENTING THE NURSING SHORTAGE

The nursing shortage, although improving, is a well-known phenomenon that continues to be a problem. Home care providers as an industry have not come to terms with the growing need for additional nurses rendering hands-on or bedside care and the continuing exacerbation of this problem over the next decade. The following factors contribute to the problem:

1. Fewer students are choosing the nursing profession.
2. Of the nursing graduates, home care is often not a viable option due to the uncontrolled environment and their lack of actual experience.
3. The elderly population is continuing to grow, which will further strain the need for more bedside nurses.

4. Experienced nurses have greater opportunities available to them outside of bedside nursing. These options include:
   - case managers for insurance companies
   - utilization review for large groups
   - administrative positions
   - management positions
   - marketing positions
   - teaching positions

The net result of these intervening variables is that as the need for bedside nursing grows, the number of available caregivers is shrinking. Figure 15–1 illustrates the nursing shortage juxtaposition with need. There are only three ways in which agencies can circumvent the growing nursing shortage:

1. Design a process by which entry-level nurses can participate in home care.
2. Enhance each nurse's productivity by reducing non-nursing functions.
3. Develop a method by which nurses can enjoy professional growth and opportunity while remaining in bedside nursing.

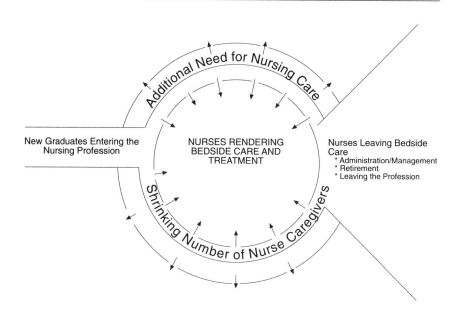

Figure 15–1 Nursing Shortage Juxtaposition with Need

Each of these evolving processes involves a commitment to staff development. The commitment must not be in the form of lip service, but rather in the form of financial support for a dedicated staff to develop, implement, and oversee the staff development program. Each of the above processes has implications:

Entry-Level Nurse Participation

The problem with new graduates or entry-level nurses is one of lack of experience in bedside nursing. Even when a nurse has been through an internship program, limited experience hampers his or her assessment and judgment skills. Additionally, these nurses have not gained the confidence level necessary to operate in an uncontrolled environment. However, home care agencies no longer have the luxury to completely exclude this group of nurses from employment.

The preceptor program can be the method by which newly graduated nurses can have a professionally rewarding experience in home care. A preceptor can be paired with two or three new graduates to oversee their work while offering the supervision and support these nurses need. Agency managers must become more creative to allow for competition in this untapped market of new nurses.

Enhanced Nurse Productivity

One of the primary complaints nurses in home care share is the burden of paperwork. It is a well-known maxim that if it isn't charted, it didn't happen. Computerized medical records do reduce the time nurses spend on charting by automating the flow of information to various forms. Charting time can be reduced by utilizing hand-held devices, and lap top or other portable computers. This time savings can be used to enhance patient care.

There are other, less obvious, duties currently performed by nurses that can be performed as easily by trained medical technicians. For example, lab results could be called into physicians' offices by a medical technician rather than the nurse. The nursing staff itself can identify many tasks that can be handled by a medical technician. Involve the nursing staff in developing a list of duties to be delegated elsewhere and allow nurses to see more patients.

Opportunities for Professional Growth in Bedside Nursing

Currently, many nurses believe that the only way they can professionally grow in home care is to accept management or supervisory positions. One group of management nurses developed a progressive approach to establishing a clinical ladder for home care.

In the clinical levels program developed by this group, nurses could progress both professionally and financially while remaining in bedside nursing. Four levels of clinical practice were identified within the framework of the clinical ladder process. The committee established education and experience criteria for the minimum standards needed to fulfill job expectations. See Figure 15–2.

Clinical Nurse I is an entry-level position for those without previous home care experience. An added benefit of this level is that it would also hold great attraction for those nurses who prefer to make home visits without the burden of

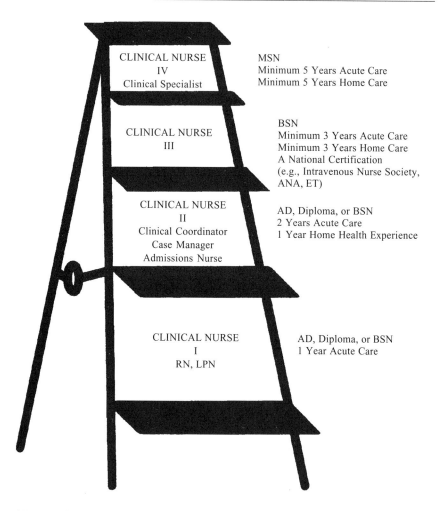

AD = associate degree; ANA = American Nurses' Association; BSN = bachelor of science in nursing; ET = enterostomal therapy; MSN = master of science in nursing.

Figure 15–2 Clinical Ladder. *Source:* Courtesy of Patricia S. Sanders, RN, Lilburn, Georgia.

additional and sometimes extensive paperwork. The nurse's responsibilities include direct patient care and supervision of home health aides (HHAs). Paperwork is limited to submission of clinical notes, physician verbal orders, and progress notes. The number of visits made daily is based on established productivity standards (35 visits per week).

Clinical Nurse II addresses the needs of the experienced home care nurse who is seeking increased responsibility and accountability in nursing practice. At this level there are three job titles: Admissions Nurse, Clinical Coordinator, and Case Manager. The Admissions Nurse's responsibilities include the assessment of new clients, development of the initial plan of care, and completion of all forms necessary for third-party reimbursement.

The Clinical Coordinator's responsibilities include primary supervision of Clinical Nurse I, management of the care rendered by the multidisciplinary field staff, and home visits prior to client recertification or discharge. Supervision of Clinical Nurse I is attained through the Clinical Coordinator's review of the medical records, on-site home visits, and weekly case conferences with the field staff.

The Case Manager functions as a primary nurse. Utilizing the nursing process, the nurse renders direct care to a defined client population and assumes the total responsibility for the coordination and management of all client care needs.

Clinical Nurse III is designed for the nurse who chooses to utilize specialized training and skills to promote staff development. The Clinical Nurse III's responsibilities are to teach, update, and validate skills of Clinical Nurse I and II. She or he acts as a preceptor and serves as a consultant to staff. In addition, the nurse conducts ongoing quality assurance surveillance, identifies educational needs, develops and presents inservices, and evaluates the effectiveness of inservices through the re-audit process. Home visits are performed to accomplish these responsibilities (15 visits per week).

Clinical Nurse IV (Clinical Specialist) was developed as an integral part of the plan to upgrade current standards of nursing practice within the agency. The Clinical Specialist demonstrates expertise achieved from years of experience and advanced education. The level IV nurse carries specialized consultative responsibilities in home health nursing and assists in the promotion and development of nursing activities in the agency. Additionally, the nurse would assist in the preparation of manuals, guidelines, and procedures related to nursing service; conduct surveillance studies and surveys; prepare reports as required; and make recommendations and improvements in service delivery to administrative and nursing staff.

This clinical levels program has the advantage of allowing nurses the freedom to move up the ladder while allowing the agency to fully utilize the expertise of nurses in their areas of specialty.

Figure 15-3 shows the percentage of budgeted nursing positions versus percentage of visits made by each clinical level. An unexpected advantage of this program for the agency that developed it was a cost savings of over $200,000. See Exhibit 15-1.

While the levels program offers many advantages to nurses and the agency alike, there is a rigorous testing component for each level. The testing is conducted by staff development to ensure clinical competence at each level before progressing to the next. The testing component includes:

1. written examination
2. oral examination
3. chart audit
4. field audit

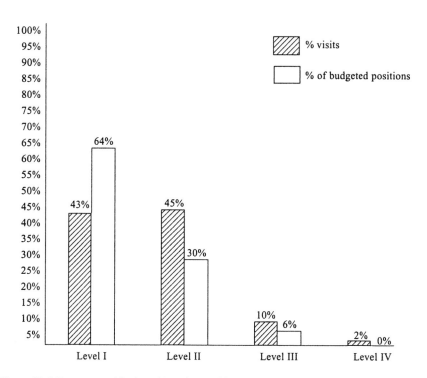

Figure 15-3 Percentage of Budgeted Nursing Positions vs. Percentage of Visits Made by Each Clinical Level. *Source:* Courtesy of Patricia S. Sanders, RN, Lilburn, Georgia.

Exhibit 15–1 Agency Budget for Allocated Nursing Positions

(Based on 1,000 Nursing Visits Per Week)		
CURRENT	*Visits*	*Salary*
Case Managers—50 RNs	1,000	$1,352,000
PROJECTED	*Visits*	*Salary*
Clinical Nurse I—18 (9 RNs/9 LPNs)	630	$ 411,830
Clinical Nurse II—9 Clinical Coordinators	90	262,080
4 Admissions Nurses	60	116,480
6 Case Managers	150	174,720
Clinical Nurse III—4	60	124,800
Clinical Nurse IV—1 Clinical Specialist	0	33,280
	990	$1,123,200
	$1,352,000	
	−1,123,200	
COST SAVINGS =	$ 228,800	

Source: Courtesy of Patricia S. Sanders, RN, Lilburn, Georgia.

THE NURSE ORIENTATION PROGRAM

Knowledge of the ways and means of retaining current nurses and opportunities to recruit new nurses is incorporated into the actual orientation objectives and training.

Nursing Orientation Objectives

The objectives of the orientation program are to provide the orientee with the information and resources needed to:

1. manage and provide quality patient care in the home setting, with consistent conformance to customer expectations, within the guidelines of agency policies and procedures and regulatory requirements
2. promote the use of nursing process to assess, plan, implement, and evaluate outcome-oriented client care reflecting the total needs of the client and family

3. complete and maintain documentation of case managed care in accordance with federal, state, and external review standards, and reflective of nursing practice
4. facilitate case-managed continuity of care incorporating inter- and intra-agency and community resources in the ongoing plan of care and in the discharge plans
5. give special consideration to appropriate interventions for and thorough documentation of high-risk clients and situations
6. perform nursing procedures specific to home care with clinical competence based on agency and professional standards of care

Day 1 RN Orientation

Objectives

After completing Day 1 of the RN orientation program, the orientee will be able to:

1. state agency personnel policies and procedures related to employment
2. describe agency philosophy and the orientee's role in achieving agency mission
3. identify services and disciplines commonly found in home health care
4. explain the philosophy and characteristics of specific programs offered by agency

Outline

The first day's orientation will cover:

1. explanation of orientation process, review of overall objectives, and review of Day 1 objectives
2. history of company to present day, including growth and agency philosophy
3. personnel forms—any pertinent personnel forms to be completed will be handed out
4. personnel policies and procedures related to the RN's employment and functioning with the agency
5. responsibilities of the employee with regard to retention of current license, CPR certification, driver's license, health maintenance, address and phone, compliance with standards
6. rights of the employee, including the agency's open door philosophy, grievance procedures, and suggestion programs

7. overview of home health
   a. reasons for growth:
      - cost savings—home care costs are 30–70 percent of hospital care
      - consumer values are changing toward caring for sick in home
      - increased number of elderly
      - changes in third-party reimbursement, such as Medicare (quicker and sicker, diagnosis-related groups [DRGs], catastrophic care extensions of benefits)
      - increase in technology for home use (oxygen, monitors, ventilators)
   b. types of services and disciplines found in home health:
      - RN, LPN, therapies, medical social worker (MSW), HHA, homemaker
      - acute, high tech, pediatric, rehab, custodial/maintenance
      - payment for home health:
        — Medicare 65 percent
        — entitlement programs such as Medicaid, community care services program
        — private insurance
        — client
   c. philosophy and mission of the agency, including focus of care, quality of care, and client satisfaction and the role of RN in meeting this goal through case management, client advocacy, coordination of services, and discharge planning for continuity

Day 2 RN Orientation

Objectives

After completing Day 2 of the RN orientation program, the orientee will be able to:

1. demonstrate the relationship of the admission process to the assessment aspect of nursing process
2. identify expected outcomes of the admission visit for the client, family, and case manager
3. integrate the nursing process and the Assessment Plan Implementation Evaluation (APIE) documentation format
4. correlate management of legal, ethical, and professional risk with specific nursing measures according to agency policy and procedure
5. identify specific documentation guidelines associated with risk management

Outline

The second day's orientation will cover:

1. a review of objectives of Day 2
2. nursing process review
   a. review of nursing process
   b. relationship of nursing process to home health care
   c. use of nursing diagnosis in home health care and diagnostic clusters for ease of finding diagnosis
   d. nursing process and the clinical record, including purposes of the record:
      - reflection of practice
      - legal document
      - assurance of quality for client
      - record of coordination of services and continuity of care
      - invoice for care
3. assessment
   a. definition—the process of obtaining comprehensive data about clients, caregivers, environment, and health status to determine appropriate nursing interventions based on desired outcome
   b. relationship of the assessment to continued nursing care
   c. start of care (SOC) visit and assessment as part of nursing process— discussion of purpose of information, including problems with incomplete or incorrect information
   d. expected outcomes of SOC visit for client and family, to include client knowledge of:
      - when to expect a nurse again
      - emergency and safety procedures relevant to care
      - how to reach agency and nurse
      - goals and plans of care (with client agreement)
   e. expected outcomes for case manager, who should have comprehensive assessment to formulate plan of care based on physical and psychosocial needs of client
4. development of care plan
   a. formulation of plan of care using assessment information (development of plan of care using theoretical client)
   b. formulation of outcome-oriented plans, working with nursing diagnosis to include:
      - expected outcomes (long-range to discharge and short-range expected visits)
      - relationship to medical and nursing diagnoses
      - measurable and attainable goals

5. nursing process and APIE charting for clinical notes
   a. assessment—subjective and objective measures
   b. plan—formulation of today's plan based on assessment from today and nursing care plan
   c. intervention—specific actions, skilled actions, and, if teaching, what was taught
   d. evaluation—response to intervention, whether next visit will be evaluated, whether last visit will be evaluated
   e. review of APIE samples
   f. timeliness of paperwork and relation to following plan of care
6. risk management
   a. patient rights and responsibilities—customer satisfaction
   b. high-risk situations—abandonment, safety, noncompliance
   c. high-risk clients—high tech, infectious diseases, AIDS
   d. documentation guidelines for risk management (handout on assumption of risk forms)
7. infection control
   a. handwashing
   b. universal precautions
   c. bag technique
   d. sharps disposal
   e. waste disposal

Days 3–5 RN Orientation

Days 3–5 of the orientation program are conducted in the field.

Objectives

After completing Day 3 of the RN orientation program, the orientee will be able to:

1. compare in-home assessment and nursing intervention to the theoretical basis of home health care
2. identify specific areas for in-home risk management
3. evaluate short- and long-term goals for clients visited

After completing Days 4 and 5 of the RN orientation program, the orientee will be able to:

1. demonstrate competence in the following procedures based on agency policy and procedure and on professional standards of care:

a. bag technique
b. handwashing
c. sharps disposal
d. dressing change
e. waste disposal
2. exhibit understanding of nursing process in documentation for:
a. clinical notes
b. care plan updating and development

Day 6 RN Orientation

Objectives

After completing Day 6 of the RN orientation program, the orientee will be able to:

1. relate admission criteria and services provided by entitlement programs for which agency is certified
2. review the American Nurses' Association standards of care for home health
3. demonstrate comprehension of the start of care process for private pay, insurance, Medicaid, community care service program
4. correlate the appropriate use of nursing process to reimbursement
5. identify community and agency resources to utilize in coordination of care and discharge planning

Outline

The sixth day's orientation will cover:

1. third-party reimbursement:
a. private insurance—national trends
b. Medicaid—eligibility and restrictions
c. community care service program—eligibility and services
d. hospice
e. Medicare—Part A and Part B
f. levels of care by reimbursement source
2. plans of treatment
a. private insurance and private pay
b. Medicaid
c. community care service program

    d. hospice
    e. other SOC forms
3. review of standards of care
    a. American Nurses' Association standards
    b. home visit audits
    c. outcome criteria
    d. coordination of services
4. community and agency resources
    a. discussion of types of additional services a client might need and how to locate them
    b. community resources/handouts:
       • United Way Help Book
       • American Cancer Society
       • Enterostomal therapy (ET), chemotherapy, pediatricians, medical social worker agency resources

Day 7 RN Orientation

Objectives

After completing Day 7 of the RN orientation program, the orientee will be able to:

1. explain conditions of coverage for Medicare, and cite examples of each condition
2. demonstrate comprehension of the start of care process for Medicare clients including use of 485, 486, and 487
3. relate the information requested on the Health Care Financing Administration (HCFA) forms to assessment, and nursing care plan information

Outline

The seventh day's orientation will cover:

1. Medicare conditions of coverage
    a. homebound, frequency and reasons for leaving home
    b. skilled, licensed person, assessment
    c. reasonable and necessary, medical and nursing diagnoses
    d. under care of physician, medical director, accessible
    e. intermittent, meaning and frequencies
    f. end stage renal disease patients

2. completion of forms (485 and 486)
   a. review information needed in each blank, correlate to assessment information and nursing care plan, and relate to quality of care and coordination of services
      - no generalized statements
      - no packaged statements
      - diagnosis specific care first
      - legibility
      - appropriate diagnosis (no symptoms or treatments)
   b. guidelines for completion
      - 486 treatment codes
      - ICD-9-CM codes
      - frequency abbreviations
3. ongoing progess record (487) and relationship to care of clinical notes and forms 485, 486
4. recertification process
   a. reassessment
   b. timeliness
   c. completion of forms—differences from start of care

Days 8–10 RN Orientation

Objectives

After completing Days 8, 9, and 10 of the RN orientation program, the orientee will be able to:

1. complete a start of care for at least two different programs utilizing nursing process
2. demonstrate clinical competence based on agency policy and procedure and professional standards of care in the following:
   a. physical assessment
   b. medication teaching and review
   c. disease-specific teaching
   d. venipuncture
3. utilize nursing process in evaluating and updating the nursing care plan

Day 11 RN Orientation

Objectives

After completing Day 11 of the RN orientation program, the orientee will be able to:

1. describe the documentation and case management responsibilities for supervision, communication, and coordination of care

Outline

The eleventh day's orientation will cover:

1. case management responsibilities
   a. coordination of care
   b. chart
2. specifics
   a. schedules and calling office
      • LPN scheduling
   b. visits—relationship to reimbursement and to nursing care plan
   c. review of progress notes
   d. verbal order process
      • change in frequency, care, medications
      • discharge—show continuity of care
   e. transfer forms
   f. referrals to ET, rehabilitation, hospice
   g. labs—location, results, calling physician
   h. change in data base
   i. on hold/hospitalizations
   j. 60 day summaries
3. end-of-month chart review
   a. recertification process review—nursing care plan update, home health aide
   b. HHA supervision (handout guidelines)
   c. team and case conferences—documentation and relationship to care
   d. coordination of therapies
   e. intra-agency communication
   f. management of supplies
      • policies
      • reimbursement
   g. discharge procedure
   h. nonadmission
   i. weekend and on-call work

Days 12–15 RN Orientation

Days 12 through 15 of the orientation program take place in the field.

Objectives

After completing Days 12 through 15 of the RN orientation program, the orientee will be able to:

1. perform home health aide supervision utilizing established criteria
2. appropriately utilize the 487 or ongoing progress record
3. show understanding of the verbal order process
4. correctly complete recertification process including plan of treatment (POT), 60-day summary
5. complete an aide assignment revision and nursing care plan update
6. follow agency procedures for management of supplies
7. exhibit clinical competence based on agency policy and procedure and professional standards of care in the care of:
   a. selected high risk patients (e.g., AIDS, noncompliance)
   b. Foley catheter patient
   c. IV patient (central line preferred)

Day 16 RN Orientation

Objectives

After completing Day 16 of the RN orientation program, the orientee will be able to:

1. correctly complete incident reports
2. identify personal needs in ongoing educational process

Outline

The sixteenth day's orientation will cover:

1. incident reports
   a. identification of root cause
2. review of start of care
   a. group input and suggestions for improvement
   b. participants share a start of care they prepared (plan of treatment, nursing care plan, assessment, etc.)
3. questions and answer line on any aspect of orientation program
4. customer satisfaction
   a. understanding expectations of clients

b. dealing with different clients
c. listening and responding
d. meeting and exceeding expectations
e. practicing social courtesy

Days 17–20 RN Orientation

Objectives

After completing Days 17 through 20 of the RN orientation program, the orientee will be able to:

1. utilize the master schedule for communicating and planning the week's work
2. incorporate intra-agency and community resources in discharge planning

Continuing Orientation

Each Monday for the next month the orientee will meet with the branch manager, the director of professional services, or the staff development director to review clinical notes, start of care, coordination of services, HHA supervision, and case management responsibilities.

Objective

Weekly meetings with management persons will provide guidance and suggestions for documentation, provision of care, and case management to allow the orientee to correct problems as they arise and to be able to function as an independent case manager.

HHA ORIENTATION

The objectives of the HHA orientation program are to provide the orientee with the information and resources needed to:

1. provide quality client care in the home setting, with consistent conformance to customer expectations, within the guidelines of agency policies and procedures and regulatory requirements
2. complete and maintain documentation in accordance with agency standards with consideration for risk management

3. perform client care procedures specific to home care with competence based on federal, state, and agency standards of care

Days 1 and 2

Days 1 and 2 of the HHA orientation follow the nursing orientation for Days 1 and 2 as they relate to the aide's discipline.

Day 3

Objectives

After completing Day 3 of the HHA orientation, the orientee will be able to:

1. delineate specific responsibilities of the HHA to the agency supervisors and clients
2. identify documentation guidelines pertinent to quality care and risk management
3. contrast basic changes associated with normal aging to abnormal changes
4. relate caregiving interventions for the HHA to assist in compensation for age-related changes
5. identify those client changes and conditions that require reporting

Outline

The third day's orientation for HHAs will cover:

1. HHA role:
   a. place on home care team
   b. supervisors
   c. getting assignments
   d. assignment sheet
   e. schedules
   f. calling clients
   g. "no show" clients
   h. in-home supervision
   i. who to call and for what
2. documentation
   a. notes compared to assignment sheet
   b. facts vs. opinions

    c. ink

    d. errors

    e. timeliness

3. communication

    a. types of communication

       • verbal

       • nonverbal

    b. communicating with older people

    c. communicating with ill people

    d. communicating with people who speak a different language

    e. communicating with deaf people

    f. importance of effective communication for HHAs

4. client assessment

    a. normal changes of aging and how the HHA's care helps to compensate

       • skin and hair

       • heart and lungs

       • bones and muscles

       • sensory organs—demonstration

       • brain—confusion

    b. symptoms of illness

       • temperature changes in the older person

       • blood pressure

       • pulse

       • respirations

       • bowel changes

       • appetite

       • hydration

       • hyper- and hypoglycemia (blood sugar)

       • what to report and to whom

       • how to document

    c. psychosocial factors

       • home environment

       • caregivers

       • abuse

5. questions and concerns

EVALUATING THE STAFF DEVELOPMENT PROGRAM

The best way to determine the effectiveness of a staff development program is to break the evaluation into its components, i.e., evaluate by the objective of the class. See Exhibit 15–2 for an example of this kind of evaluation.

Exhibit 15–2 Sample Post-Orientation Evaluation

How effective was this program in teaching you to:	EXCELLENT	GOOD	FAIR	POOR	NOT AT ALL
1. State agency personnel policies and procedures related to employment.					
2. Describe agency philosophy and the orientee's role in achieving agency mission.					
3. Identify services and disciplines commonly found in home health care.					
4. Explain the philosophy and specific characteristics of the hospice program.					

For general topics, a standard evaluation tool will suffice. It is important that all staff members have an opportunity to request an inservice or program that would be beneficial to their individual needs. Agencies should attempt to provide inservices as requested by the staff.

STAFF RECRUITMENT AND SELECTION

Although this chapter deals with staff development, the issue of recruitment and selection of staff is too important to ignore. Recruiting appropriate staff for home care is not as simple as for an institution where everyone is in a supervised setting. Since home care is largely an independent practice, the staff members must be able to function appropriately in an uncontrolled environment.

There is a race among providers to secure the best staff available. Recruitment relies on job fairs, schools, advertising locally and nationally, other health care providers, professional associations, and word of mouth. Of these, word of mouth is the most effective. Nurses like to work for a company where other nurses are happy and enjoying their work.

Selection of Staff

Selection of new staff should follow a rigorous process to ensure, insofar as possible, that only appropriate staff members are allowed to represent the agency. The selection process should begin with a basic skills test to determine the level of competence of the potential candidate for hire. Because of home care's growth rate and the shortage of nurses, agencies will have a tendency to accept applicants who score in the middle to low range rather than only those in the high range. This is a dangerous attitude for the following reasons:

1. The prehire test is a *minimum* skills test.
2. Nurses working in an uncontrolled environment with little hands-on supervision should have *better than average* skills for the safety and welfare of patients.
3. Nurses with low basic skills will create a higher risk for agencies.
4. The top of the class nurses will not want to be associated with agencies that build in mediocrity by design.
5. This attitude is not in keeping with the process of offering the best possible service with continuous improvements.

Agencies that are considering reducing the passing percentage on the basic skills test should be warned to avoid the tendency toward self-deception. The agency is a direct reflection of the competence of the staff.

After competency and licensure have been validated, the agency should use extreme caution in handling reference checks. References should be checked at as many former places of employment as possible, but a minimum of three where the duties were the same or similar. In other words, it does no good to validate experience in a job unrelated to the one for which employment is being sought. For example, a nursing assistant who gives three references from fast food restaurants and a car wash does little for your feeling of comfort regarding this person's ability to effectively deal with patients, even if the candidate was a recent graduate from a training program for nursing assistants.

Because of the safety factor, many agencies are doing criminal checks on applicants before hire. This is a good idea if it is appropriate in your state. Agency administrators have a fiduciary responsibility to protect the safety and welfare of patients insofar as possible. The issue of appropriate screening of potential candidates for hire should never be taken lightly.

JOINT COMMISSION REQUIREMENTS

The Joint Commission on Accreditation of Healthcare Organizations (Joint Commission) requires that the agency staff members participate in orientation and inservice programming. The following summarizes the Joint Commission requirements:

- Orientation is provided prior to staff seeing patients.
- Orientation includes:
  —service delivery in the home

—community resources
—safety and equipment management
—infection control
—confidentiality
—actions in unsafe situations
—policies and procedures
- Inservice programming provided is appropriate to the needs of staff.
—There is evidence that staff attends all programming.
—The number, qualifications, and competence of individuals providing care are appropriate to meet patient needs.
—Supervision of services and staff is appropriate.
—A consistent process is used for the selection of support service staff.
—Processes are defined in policy to cover reference checks, interviews, job history, and education.
—Staff demonstrates proficiency with assigned responsibilities.

THE SUCCESSFUL STAFF DEVELOPMENT PROGRAM

The ultimate successes of the staff development program will be apparent throughout the agency's operations. A successful staff development program will be evidenced by:

- improved client outcomes as evidenced by improved results in diagnosis-related and other audits
- improved conformance with standards of compliance, i.e., federal, state, and Joint Commission
- improved patient, client, and employee satisfaction
- improved staff turnover rates
- improved efficiency and productivity

Staff development is not cheap. Agencies with a real commitment to quality cannot afford the luxury of being without someone dedicated to this most important function. As a wise man once said, "A leader is one who sees the need for change when things are going well."

Staff development is a continuous process as new people are hired and as current employees want to excel in their profession. Under the continuous quality improvement process, staff development becomes the manner in which resolution is found to all problems associated with special cause variations. Additionally, almost every employee will need to be trained in the concepts and methods of continuous quality improvement. Education and training is the agency's commitment to the future.

Glossary

Administrative Review—A review of any nonclinical function for which specific quantifiable measures have been set and can be either process or outcome in focus.

Aspects of Care—Relates to the patient and should be focused on standards of care.

Attributes Control Charts—Attributes are derived from counts. Control charts using attributes data will usually be bimodal in distribution. Effective charts from this type of data are the p chart and the np chart.

Average and Range Charts—The $\bar{X}$ and R charts are used for variables data with a normal distribution.

Bag Technique—A method by which infection control precautions can be maintained by those who use nursing or other bags in the home care setting.

Bell-Shaped Curve—A statistical method establishing the shape of a normal distribution of data approximating the shape of a bell. Once data has attained this shape, other statistical tests can be applied.

Bimodal Distribution—A distribution of data that has two dominant peaks. This shape will generally occur with attributes data. Because the distribution is not normal, certain statistical formulas must be applied to developing control charts.

Brainstorming—The art of allowing a free flow of ideas without restriction; allows for enhanced creativity.

Cause and Effect Diagram—Commonly called the fishbone diagram, this tool is designed to distinguish cause from effect and is a good tool for the determination of root causes.

CDCP—The Centers for Disease Control and Prevention in Atlanta, Georgia.

Central Limit Theorem—A statistical methodology that allows data to be manipulated into a normal distribution using the measures of central limit (mean, medium, and mode).

Client Advocate—One designated to speak on behalf of patients. In the context of this book, the advocate is generally the utilization review (UR) nurse, who will be attempting to gain appropriate coverage for patients under private insurance or could argue for continued coverage under Medicare if a denial has been made.

Client Satisfaction Index—A measurable way of determining trends in customer service. The index is used in conjunction with a quantifiable questionnaire.

Clinical Ladder—A method by which nurses can have advancement opportunity without leaving bedside nursing.

Collection Period Ratio—A mathematically calculated ratio to determine the average number of days it takes to collect accounts receivable.

Common Cause Variation—Variation caused from the process itself. Only management can improve common causes by improving the system.

Concurrent—A timing sequence that refers to current period.

Conformance to Requirements—A simplified definition of quality.

Continuous Quality Improvement (CQI)—A system that relies on statistical methods to stabilize, control, and improve processes. This system is management led and customer focused.

Control Charts—The tools used to determine whether processes are stable and in control.

Control Limits—Limits that are set using a statistical formula; considered the voice of the process.

Correlation—A correlation is seen when two variables are related to each other.

Crosby, Philip—A quality guru best known for his work with the concept of zero defects.

Customers—Anyone upstream or downstream in a process, but the focus for quality is always the end user. Types of customers:

- Primary: end users or those who order end use
- Secondary: payers and regulators
- Auxiliary: employees, contractors, and stockholders

Data Collection—A systematic process to gather data necessary for surveillance or audit purposes.

Data Element—A specific fact or piece of information.

Data Source—A planned, articulated, and consistent place to find specific data elements.

Defect Location Diagram—A visualization of the location of problems.

Deming, Edwards W.—Some call him the father of quality. He was the first to articulate the statistical basis for quality and is best known for his 14 management points.

Deploy—The process of implementation.

Design—The manner in which to construct a process, audit, or program.

Diagnosis-Related Audits—A method by which outcome indicators can be tied to both standards of care and standards of practice.

Downstream Customer—The customer immediately after the process or the one to whom the process output is given.

Employee Exposure Categories—A means to identify the potential risk to and training in prevention for infection control by employee group.

Engineering Controls—Used in the context of this book, these controls are those that are designed into the system or process that will allow quality controls.

Entitlement Programs—Those federally mandated programs that have their basis in statutory law.

External Review Organization—Any organization that reviews other organizations by a stated set of criteria.

Field Review—An audit type that ascertains the employee's levels of compliance with technical procedures, infection control, and the patient's level of understanding after instruction.

Fishbone Diagrams—Cause and effect analysis.

Frequency Distribution—A statistical term relating to the shape of data as determined by a histogram.

Governing Body—The legally responsible group for the agency.

Grievance—A complaint by either a patient or employee.

Histogram—A statistical tool for the determination of the shape of data.

Incident Reports—A method by which data can be recorded regarding an adverse occurrence or a potential problem.

Indicators—Relate to the caregiver and are considered standards of practice.

Infection Control—A process whereby universal precautions are utilized to control the spread of and prevent future infections.

Inspections—A process where work output is reviewed to ensure standards have been met.

Internalized—The learning and continuous use of imparted information.

International Standards Organization (ISO)—A homogeneous affiliation of nations of the world for the purpose of defining international standards of quality.

ISO 9000–9004 Series—The international standards of quality.

Joint Commission 10-Step Process—The process of quality assurance as articulated by the Joint Commission on Accreditation of Healthcare Organizations.

Juran, Joseph—One of the quality gurus. Best known for the Juran Trilogy: quality planning, quality control, and quality improvement.

Key Indicators—Those standards of practice that are most important to the outcome.

Malcolm Baldrige National Quality Award—An annual award given to the companies that best exemplify the methods of continuous quality improvement.

Maslow's Hierarchy—A theory of motivation based on unmet needs of the individual.

Mean—A measure of the Central Limit Theory that is the average of a given set of numbers.

Measurement—A quantifiable identification of some element of doing business.

Medical Records Administration—A systematic means of effectively managing medical records and related functions.

Medium—A measure of the Central Limit Theorem that means the mid-point of a given set of numbers.

Mission Statement—The underlying value and principles of the company.

Monitoring—A system of processes, surveillance, or auditing to determine problem identification or areas where improvements can be initiated.

Moving Averages—A statistical process to assist in averaging large numbers in a set.

Moving Ranges—A statistical process to assist in finding the ranges in a large data set.

Normal Distribution—Data that approximates a bell shape. Normal distribution is necessary to calculate standard deviations.

np Chart—A statistical formula applied to attributes data to allow control charting.

Occurrence Ratio—A mathematical calculation to determine the ratio of incidents to an unduplicated census count.

Operational Definition—The specific step-by-step procedure of any process. Definitions should include quantifiable measures and establish criteria for "good versus bad."

Outcome—The end result of any process.

Outcome Audits—Those that validate that the care rendered had the desired results.

Outcome Indicators—Standards that validate results have desired outcomes.

Outlier—A data point that falls outside a given set of parameters.

Out of Control—A statistical determination of data that have been plotted on a control chart. Data points outside of three standard deviations are out of control.

Overlearned Skills—Skills so consistently used that thinking about the process is unnecessary.

p Chart—A mathematical formula used to develop a control chart for attributes data.

Paradigm—A mind set.

Parameter—Limits within which decisions can be made.

Pareto Chart—A statistical tool used to separate the trivial many from the vital few.

Peer Review—Can be conducted by an external review organization (e.g., peer review organization [PRO]) or can be an internal review conducted by utilization review or field review.

Performance Standards—Levels set by management that are predetermined to be acceptable.

Preceptor—A person who has been systematically trained to teach others in an on-the-job-training program.

Proactive—To cause action to occur before necessary.

Process Audits—These audits generally are administrative in nature and cover the scope of how events happen.

Process Indicators—Indicators that are within the control of the nurse or other employee being audited.

Productivity—Total work output divided by total work input.

Quality—Consistent conformance to customer expectations with minimal variation.

Quality Assurance (QA)—A system of surveillance to ensure key quality indicators are being met. Quality assurance is a back-end function.

Quality Continuation—A system by which employees can judge their own performance by known standards. This is a proactive function and is performed concurrently utilizing statistical process control.

Quality Control—A system by which standards and operational definitions necessary to meet those standards are deployed to all staff.

Quality Discipline—The technical and professional aspects of quality.

Quality Improvement—A systematic method of improving all systems and processes that is management led and customer focused. Its basis is statistical process control.

Quality Management—The total quality management program.

Rate-Based—Used in conjunction with relative rate indicators; frequent events that will necessitate trending to identify systematic problems.

Record Tracking—A system used in medical records administration to locate medical records.

Regression Analysis—A statistical analysis that compares variables to determine whether any are correlated.

Retrospective—To look at events in the past.

Risk Analysis—A determination of potential risks.

Risk Control—A systematic method to contain risks.

Risk Financing—A method to accrue funding to service any debt as a result of incurred risks.

Risk Manager—The person responsible for overseeing the risk prevention and control program.

Run Charts—A statistical tool to visually display data. Run charts will readily identify trends.

Scatter Diagram—Data points plotted on a diagram using two variables to show whether any correlation exists.

Scope—The parameters of an event. All issues to be covered within a specified context.

SENIC Project—A study conducted by CDCP that revealed that infection control was only effective with a surveillance program.

Sentinel Event—A rare and significant occurrence that warrants investigation for each event.

Service Audits—Surveillance events that cover a specific discipline.

Special Cause Variations—Variations in a process that are caused by individual actions. These special causes will fall outside the control limits of a stable process and can be identified from a variables control chart.

Specification Limits—Those limits imposed by the customer. These limits can be shown on a control chart *with control limits* but should not be confused with control limits. Specification limits are the voice of the customer.

Specifiers—Any individual or group that imposes rules, regulations, or any other condition under which an agency must operate.

Staff Development—A process to train, educate, and offer professional growth opportunities to staff. Staff development is a key quality characteristic to continuous quality improvement.

Standard Deviation—A statistical calculation from the medium of a normal distribution. Referred to as sigma.

Standards of Care—Nationally recognized standards for rendering treatments and interventions based on specific conditions.

Standards of Performance—Considered the thresholds, these are company set.

Standards of Practice—Considered the process indicators, these are the generally accepted standards under which professional practice occurs.

Statistical Process Control—The systematic control and improvement of processes utilizing statistical control methods.

Statistical Tools—Tools utilized to identify, resolve, and continuously improve quality.

Structure Indicators—Those indicators that pertain to policies, procedures, or other issues outside the control of the nurse or other individual.

Surveillance—A technique to monitor the quality program.

Team Building—A process to bring about synergy, i.e., the total group is better than any single individual.

Thresholds—Considered the performance standards, these are company set.

Total Quality Management (TQM)—The totality of the quality system.

Transformation—The changes a company or person goes through to implement continuous quality improvement.

Trending—The process of identifying patterns in data sets.

Universal Precautions—Those precautions that will prevent and control the spread of infections.

Upstream Customer—The customer that immediately precedes the process or the one that provided the process input.

Utilization Review (UR)—A peer review process to determine compliance with payer guidelines and efficient utilization of services.

Validity—Having basis in fact.

Variable—Different issues or sets of data.

Variables Data—Data that are measured.

Variation—The enemy of quality. Differences inherent in any process. The goal is to limit variation to improve quality.

Visualization—A powerful tool to see the process, problem, or opportunity to improve.

Voice of the Customer—Specification limits.

Voice of the Process—Control limits.

Waste Costs—Those costs that can be associated with lack of quality.

Workers' Compensation Loss Ratio—A mathematical formula identifying the ratio of workers' compensation costs to total gross wages.

Index

examples of suggestions and responses, 80
Superstar chart, 81, 82

T

Teams, 33–34
  basics of team membership, 33
  and flowcharting, 33–34
  writing of operational definitions, 34–35
Technical Assistance Research Programs, 104
Telephone call–back system, 91
Third party payers
  audit form for, 251
  utilization review questions, 250, 252
Thought process, 126–128
  conscious thought, 127
  subconscious thought, 128
Thresholds
  in branch audit, 300–301
  in quality assurance and improvement
    plan, 147
  usefulness of, 147
Time study, 132–134
  areas of study, 132
  managerial actions following, 133–134
  record in, 135
  study methodology in, 132–133
Total quality management, 61–70
  compared to continuous quality
    management, 62
  education in, 66–68
  example in, 67–68
  future view of, 68, 70
  nature of, 61–62
  policy in, 63–66
Tracking system, for medical records, 310
Training
  education in total quality management,
    66–68
  in infection control, 276
  on the job training, 66, 67
Trending, 295–296
  example of use, 295
Two-factor theory, 75
  motivation, 129–130

U

Universal precautions, infection control, 263
Utilization review audits, 170–172
  importance of, 247
  judgment call in, 171
  legal aspects, 253–254
  Medicare
    audit form for, 248
    utilization review questions, 249–250
  and patient advocacy, 252–253
  third party payers
    audit form for, 251
    utilization review questions, 250, 252
  time factors in, 170, 171
  trends related to, 253
  UR nurse, role of, 247, 249, 253

V

Value
  factors in determination of, 103
  value added features of service, 75–76
  value of service and price, 76–77
Value analysis, 14–15, 58–59
  purpose of, 14
  steps in process, 58–59
Variables, in statistics, 39
Variation, 45–46
  abnormal variation, 45–46, 46
  normal variation, 45, 46
Visualization, and excellence, 136

W

Waste costs, 58–60
  categories of, 58
  and value analysis, 58–59
Worker's compensation, loss ratio, 293–294

X

X Bar chart, 49